THE GAMES CELLS PLAY
Basic Concepts of Cellular Metabolism

D1300178

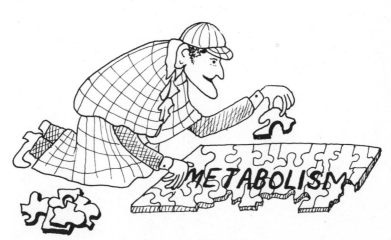

"Elementary, my dear..."

THE GAMES CELLS PLAY
Basic Concepts of Cellular Metabolism

MAX D. LECHTMAN

BONITA ROOHK

ROBERT J. EGAN

Golden West College
Huntington Beach, California

The Benjamin/Cummings Publishing Company, Inc.
Menlo Park, California • Reading, Massachusetts
London • Amsterdam • Don Mills, Ontario • Sydney

We wish to dedicate this book to our respective families: Dale, Alex, Jay, and Risa; Vern; and Ann, Katie, Chris, and Michael. In addition we wish to dedicate this book to the memory of Ruth Rodney, one who particularly loved word games.

Library of Congress Cataloging in Publication Data

Lechtman, Max D
   The games cells play.

   Includes index.
    1.   Cell metabolism.   I.   Roohk, Bonita, 1948-   joint author.
II.   Egan, Robert J., 1941-   joint author.   III.   Title.
QH634.5.L42   574.8'761   78-57373
ISBN 0-8053-6094-8

ISBN 0-8053-6094-8
CDEFGHIJKL-AL-89876543210

The Benjamin/Cummings Publishing Company, Inc.
2727 Sand Hill Road
Menlo Park, California 94025

Preface

Many students who are exposed to the study of metabolism without "reasonable" background in chemistry are mystified by the seemingly obscure terms and relationships. As instructors in Junior College–Community College programs, we sense the pain and frustration of the students but refuse to eliminate metabolism from the courses, since a knowledge of the physical and chemical changes that occur in living things is fundamental to life.

Sherlock Holmes was chosen as a symbol for this book for he is a master in taking seemingly obscure bits of information and transforming them into readily understandable stories. He resolves intricate mysteries with such ease that they become a game. Thus we have the book, *The Games Cells Play*. In this book, assuming the readers' minimal knowledge, the authors present clues to show the intermeshed workings of metabolism according to what we consider to be a reasonable game plan.

This book was written for students in the Allied Health Sciences with minimal background in the chemistry and biology of metabolism. It is a supplemental text for students in Anatomy and Physiology, Microbiology, General Biology, Zoology, and Cell Biology in the junior and community colleges. Some previous exposure to basic biology and chemistry would be helpful but not required for the use of this book

This book is divided into four sections. Section One, Rules of the Game, describes the laws obeyed in the composition and interaction of molecules. Section Two, The Players, introduces the major players in our game, that is, the basic elements, water and four kinds of organic molecules: protein, carbohydrate, lipid, and nucleic acid. Section Three, The Playing Field, describes the general structure and selected activities of the cell. Lastly, Section Four, The Game, contains a discussion of various aspects of metabolism, that is, catabolism, energy, protein synthesis, and control of enzyme activity.

Within each section, the chapters are preceded by instructional objectives to organize and focus your attention on the material to be mastered. At the end of each section is a self test to help you evaluate your progress. Answers will be found in the appendix. The glossary includes biological and chemical terms defined in the context of the material presented in this book.

We would especially like to thank Paula McKenzie for her development of the art concepts used in this book and for her expert art. We also extend our thanks to Evanelle Towne and Joel Goldstein for their art. We wish to express our sincere thanks for the helpful reviews by our colleague at GWC, Mark Souto, and allied health students Jan McNeill, Bobi Keenan, and Betty Lyons. In addition we would like to express our gratitude to the following lovely people for their typing skills: Ruth Rodney, Sharion Vandor, Susan Weins, Denise Clark, Patty Bloeser, and Thuy Tran.

Max D. Lechtman
Bonita Roohk
Robert J. Egan

Contents

THE GAMES CELLS PLAY
Basic Concepts of Cellular Metabolism

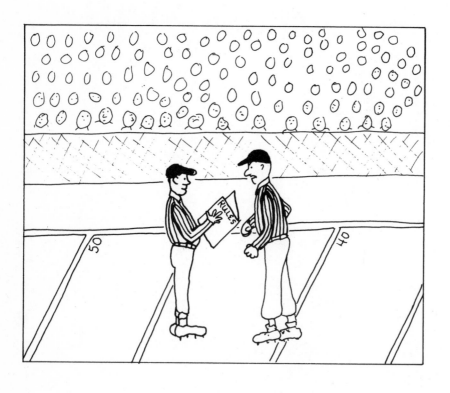

Section One
RULES OF
THE GAME

OBJECTIVES FOR SECTION ONE

Chapter 1
THE BASICS: Atoms and Molecules

1. Define terms that describe the basic units of matter including atoms, elements, molecules, and compounds.
2. Identify structural similarities and differences of all kinds of atoms.
3. Describe the different kinds of bonds that can occur between atoms and molecules.
4. Define the terms oxidation and reduction.
5. Distinguish between structural and molecular formulas.
6. Identify the components of an equation.

Chapter 2
MORE BASICS: Acids and Bases

1. Describe the importance of hydrogen ion to living systems.
2. Define the terms acid and base (alkali).
3. Describe the relationship of hydrogen ion and hydroxyl ion in an aqueous solution.
4. Use the pH scale to identify degrees of acidity or alkalinity and/or relative concentrations of hydrogen and hydroxyl ion in a solution.
5. Differentiate between strong and weak acids and bases with respect to their general pH range and their ability to neutralize a given amount of acid or base.
6. Define a buffer.
7. List common buffers in living systems and describe how each works.

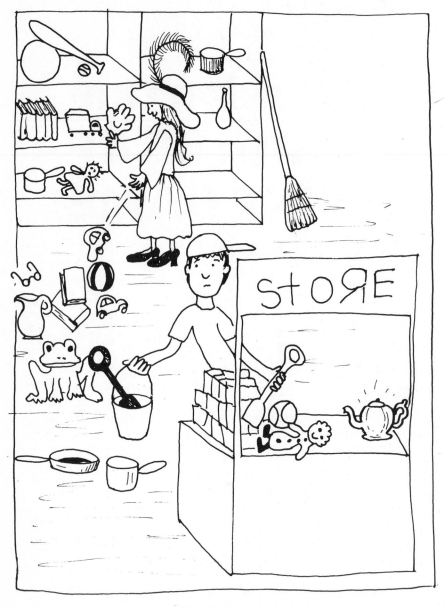

FIGURE 1–1
GAME OF STORE

Chapter 1
THE BASICS
Atoms and Molecules

WITHDRAWN

Survival to a cell is a series of "games" that must be played and won. Perhaps the game most fundamental to survival is the child's game of "store" (see Figure 1–1). In this game of make-believe, a child collects things from his or her environment such as dresses and shoes from mom, ties and shirts from dad, and cans and utensils from the kitchen. These materials are used in either of two ways. The child may modify the item for his or her own use, shortening a dress or stuffing paper in the toes of a pair of shoes; or the child may trade the materials back to the environment in exchange for something more useful like a friend's father's belt. In either case, the constant exchange of materials between the child and the environment is essential for the game to proceed. A similar, constant exchange of materials between a cell and its nonliving environment is vital to the survival of the cell.

MATTER AND ITS COMPOSITION

In order to exchange materials between a living and a nonliving environment, the environments must have a common unit exchange that is useful to both. In the case of a cell and its environment, tiny bits of matter are exchanged. In order to understand this exchange we must first define matter and describe its basic composition.

MATTER *Matter* here on earth is defined as anything that occupies space and has weight. It is the proper name for what we think of as material or substance. An ancient Greek philosopher named Democritus pondered the nature of matter and originated the concept of an *atom,* the basic unit of all matter. Democritus used the word *atomos,* which means indivisible. He reasoned that any sizable portion of matter may be divided into two smaller portions and that each of those portions may be divided and divided again. Finally a portion would remain that could no longer be divided, an indivisible portion. This portion would be the basic unit of matter, the atom.

Democritus also philosophized about the nature of the different kinds of matter. Obviously, the world is composed of more than one kind of substance. Democritus proposed that there were relatively few kinds of atoms. All other kinds of matter would be formed by various combinations of atoms.

ELEMENTS AND COMPOUNDS Although Democritus was wrong about many specifics, like the exact number and kinds of atoms, his general concepts of the nature of matter were amazingly accurate. The atom is basically as he conceived it, a unit indivisible by normal chemical means.* To date, 106 different kinds of atoms have been identified. These are called *elements* because of their simple composition. Any matter formed by the combining of two or more elements is called a *compound.* This compound exhibits different properties than those of its component elements. It becomes an entirely different form of matter.

The relationship between a compound and the elements that compose it can in some ways be compared to a manufactured product and the materials that compose it. For example, a football is an object with identifiable characteristics and properties (see Figure 1–2). It has an oval shape, is very resilient, with characteristic firmness, and is relatively lightweight. It is these properties that permit it to be kicked or thrown over 50 yards at a time.

The football represents a compound. The "elements" composing this compound, four pieces of leather, one rubber air bladder, and leather laces, all have different properties than the "compound" they combine to form. Leather, laces, or an air bladder alone cannot be kicked or thrown a significant distance. Similarly a compound has entirely different properties or characteristics than those of the elements that compose it.

Just as elements may be found in large or small amounts, so may compounds be found in variable amounts. Elements may be divided and redivided until only one of that kind of atom remains. In our football analogy, a box full of laces represents an element and one lace of that element is an atom. A box full of air bladders is another element that is composed of individual atoms. The atom, therefore, is the basic unit, the smallest unit, of an element. Similarly, a compound, like a room full of

---

*Although special techniques first developed during World War II led to the splitting of the atom and the "nuclear age," these methods are not found in living systems and will not be considered in this book.

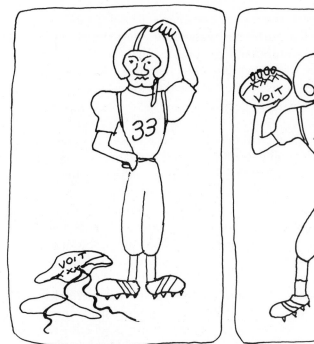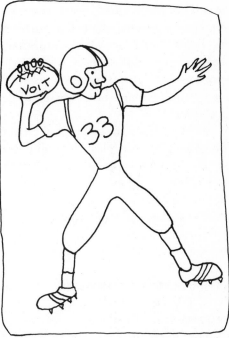

FIGURE 1-2
BEFORE AND AFTER: ELEMENTS AND COMPOUND

footballs, may be divided and redivided until only one unit of that compound remains, one football. This basic unit of a compound is a *molecule*. Just as a football may be split into laces, leather, and an air bladder, a molecule can be split further by ordinary chemical means into the atoms that compose it. What remains, however, is atoms of the various elements that composed the compound. The compound itself, the football, is now gone. Thus, a molecule is the smallest unit of a compound that still retains the properties of that compound.

Water is an example of a compound. Like all compounds it can be found in variable amounts: oceans full, pitchers full, glasses full. The smallest unit of water, however, is one molecule. An atom of water does not exist, because when a water molecule is split into its component atoms, elements appear. In this case, two atoms of the element hydrogen and one atom of the element oxygen result. Hydrogen and oxygen have entirely different properties from each other and from water. For example, neither one is a liquid at normally occuring atmospheric temperatures and pressures.

All matter, from both living and nonliving things, is composed of compounds and elements. It is the basic units of these compounds and elements, namely molecules and atoms, that the shopkeeper cell trades with its environment. In general, the cell acquires molecules containing the elements it requires to build its own structures and perform its own functions. It breaks these supplied molecules down into the component atoms and rearranges these atoms into new useful molecules. The atoms it does not need, it reorganizes into "waste" molecules, which it "trades" back to the environment.

Throughout the remaining chapters of this book we will be describing this game that cells play. We will describe the kinds of elements required by cells, the molecules they are forming that distinguish them from their environment, and even the "moves" they must execute in order to form these molecules and win the game. As with all games, however, to understand the play you must first know the rules. To understand how and why atoms combine as they do, you must first know the structure of an atom and the rules by which it combines.

ATOMIC STRUCTURE   All atoms are composed of two identifiable regions, a dense, centrally located *nucleus* and a surrounding space that is a vacuum except for the relatively few particles it contains that orbit the nucleus. There are three kinds of particles distributed within these two regions (see Figure 1–3). The two heaviest particles are located within the dense nucleus. One of these, called a *proton,* has a positive electrical charge. The other, called a *neutron,* is neutral, meaning it has no electrical charge. The third kind of particle, the *electron,* is the light particle found revolving around the nucleus within definite regions called *energy levels.* Except for the electrons they contain, the energy levels are regions of empty space.

The electron is so light in weight that we consider its weight insignificant in comparison to the weights of the neutron and proton, each of which has been given the arbitrary weight of approximately one dalton.* The electron's electrical charge, however, is a negative one. It exactly opposes the single positive charge of a proton, so that one proton and one electron together are neutral; they exactly counter each other. The lightness of the electron allows it to revolve around the nucleus within the energy levels at incredible speeds (approximately the speed of light). Its negative charge, however, causes it to be attracted by the positive nucleus so it does not fly free of the atom and become separated.

DIFFERENCES BETWEEN ELEMENTS   Each of the 106 different kinds of atoms has this same basic structure. The elements differ only in the number of particles composing their atoms. The element is determined by the number of protons it contains. This number is so significant, it is given

---

*A unit of mass approximately equal to 1.67×10^{-24} grams.

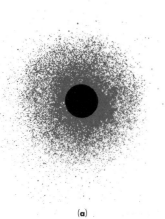

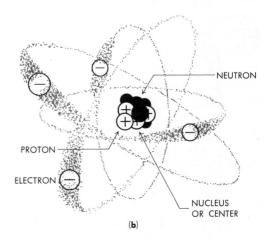

(a) (b)

FIGURE 1-3

(A) THE MODERN CONCEPTION OF THE ATOM,
SHOWING THE DENSE, CENTRALLY LOCATED NU-
CLEUS AND THE OUTER HAZE OF ELECTRONS.
(B) DIAGRAMMATIC SKETCH OF THE ATOM SHOW-
ING ITS PARTS. NEGATIVELY CHARGED ELECTRONS
CIRCLE THE NUCLEUS OF PROTONS AND NEUTRONS.
THIS DIAGRAM REPRESENTS A WORKING MODEL OF
THE ATOM. IT DOES NOT, IN ANY REAL SENSE,
REPRESENT A PICTURE OF THE ATOM. Baker and Allen,
Matter, Energy and Life, 3rd edition, p. 95.

a special name, the *atomic number*. This number alone will identify the
element. For example, all atoms with atomic number one have only one
proton, and they are all hydrogen. Similarly, all atoms with atomic number six have six protons, and they are all carbon.

Part a of Figure 1–4 is of the periodic table of elements. It is a roster
of players with the elements listed in order of increasing atomic number
when read across. Part b of the same figure shows the information given
about an element by each square of that table. The atomic number seven
identifies the element as having seven protons. The knowledgeable fan is
aware that all atoms begin play with no net electrical charge because the
number of protons and electrons are equal. Therefore, the kind of atom
shown also has seven electrons.

Because the roster lists elements, each position on the roster must
represent a team of like players. For example, all hydrogen atoms are on
hydrogen's team and oxygen atoms are on oxygen's team. The elements
are somewhat like 106 different "tag-teams" at a wrestling tournament
(see Figure 1–5). Each team has its own properties or role to play (good
guys, bad guys, underdogs, and so on). All the players of a tag-team fill
the same role. Thus, all members of a team, like atoms of an element, are
interchangeable.

(a)

PERIODIC TABLE OF THE ELEMENTS

	IA	IIA	IIIB	IVB	VB	VIB	VIIB		VIIIB
1	1 H 1.008								
2	3 Li 6.941	4 Be 9.012							
3	11 Na 22.990	12 Mg 24.305							
4	19 K 39.102	20 Ca 40.08	21 Sc 44.956	22 Ti 47.90	23 V 50.941	24 Cr 51.996	25 Mn 54.938	26 Fe 55.847	27 Co 58.933
5	37 Rb 85.468	38 Sr 87.62	39 Y 88.906	40 Zr 91.22	41 Nb 92.906	42 Mo 95.94	43 Tc 98.602	44 Ru 101.07	45 Rh 102.905
6	55 Cs 132.905	56 Ba 137.34	57 La 138.905	72 Hf 178.49	73 Ta 180.948	74 W 183.85	75 Re 186.2	76 Os 190.2	77 Ir 192.22
7	87 Fr (223)	88 Ra 226.02	89 Ac (227)	104	105				

58 Ce 140.12	59 Pr 140.907	60 Nd 144.24	61 Pm (145)	62 Sm 150.4	63 Eu 151.96	64 Gd 157.25	65 Tb 158.925	66 Dy 162.50
90 Th 232.038	91 Pa 231.036	92 U 238.029	93 Np 237.048	94 Pu (244)	95 Am (243)	96 Cm (247)	97 Bk (247)	98 Cf (251)

FIGURE 1-4

(A) PERIODIC TABLE OF THE ELEMENTS
(B) INFORMATION GIVEN ABOUT AN ELEMENT

VIIIB	IB	IIB	IIIA	IVA	VA	VIA	VIIA	Noble gases
								2 He 4.003
			5 B 10.81	6 C 12.011	7 N 14.007	8 O 15.999	9 F 18.998	10 Ne 20.179
			13 Al 26.982	14 Si 28.086	15 P 30.974	16 S 32.06	17 Cl 35.453	18 Ar 39.948
28 Ni 58.71	29 Cu 63.546	30 Zn 65.37	31 Ga 69.72	32 Ge 72.59	33 As 74.922	34 Se 78.96	35 Br 79.904	36 Kr 83.80
46 Pd 106.4	47 Ag 107.868	48 Cd 112.40	49 In 114.82	50 Sn 118.69	51 Sb 121.75	52 Te 127.60	53 I 126.905	54 Xe 131.30
78 Pt 195.09	79 Au 196.966	80 Hg 200.59	81 Tl 204.37	82 Pb 207.19	83 Bi 208.2	84 Po (~210)	85 At ~210	86 Rn (~222)

67 Ho 164.930	68 Er 167.26	69 Tm 168.934	70 Yb 173.04	71 Lu 174.97
99 Es (254)	100 Fm (257)	101 Md (256)	102 No (254)	103 Lr (257)

(b)

7 ---- Atomic number = Protons = Electrons

N ---- Atomic symbol

14.007 -- Atomic weight = Protons plus neutrons (or mass)

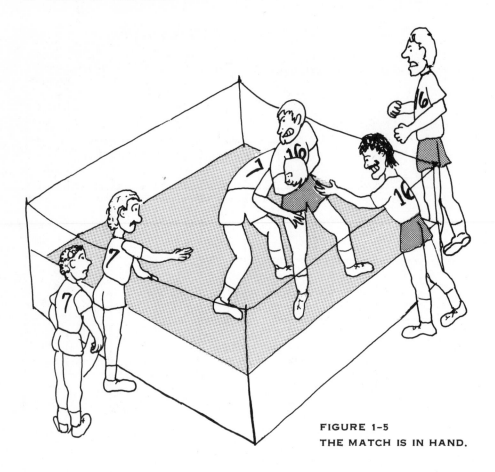

FIGURE 1-5
THE MATCH IS IN HAND.

ISOTOPES AND ATOMIC WEIGHT Just as the individual members of a wrestling tag-team may differ in weight without it altering their identity, so can the atoms of one element differ in weight. These atoms of the same element that have different weights are called *isotopes* of each other.

The existence of isotopes creates a problem for the jersey maker in our game. There is a second number associated with each tag-team or element in the tournament, its *atomic weight.* Since each element or team has member atoms of different weights, this number represents their average weight. Because the average weight of our example element is 14.007, we know that most members of this element probably weigh 14, but that there are a few who weigh more—perhaps 15 or even 16.

Atomic weight is determined by the number of weighted particles in the atom, chiefly protons plus neutrons. Recall that electrons have insignificant weight for our purposes. Since the proton number determines the player's identity, it may not change. Weight differences within an element, therefore, are due to differences in the number of neutrons present in the nucleus. Atoms of our example element with an atomic weight of 14 have 7 protons and 7 neutrons. Those atoms with a weight of 15 still have 7 protons, but this time, they possess 8 neutrons. They are isotopes of each other.

ATOMIC SYMBOLS There is one more part to our player's jersey in Part b of Figure 1–4, the letter N. This is the *atomic symbol,* and it represents the name of our element, nitrogen. Atomic symbols consist of one or two letters. The first letter is always capitalized, the second, if present, is always lower case, and there is never a space between letters (see Table 1–1). Many atomic symbols are easy to recognize because they are the first letter of the element's name. For example, C represents carbon, O represents oxygen, P is for phosphorus, H is for hydrogen, and S is for sulfur. The second lower case letter is needed when the first letter has already been used for another element. For example, calcium cannot use C because that is the symbol for carbon; instead, calcium is Ca. A lower case second letter is used so as not to confuse the second letter "a" with another element with a symbol of "A." In still other cases, the atomic symbol has been derived from the Latin name for the element. For example, sodium cannot use the symbol S or potassium the symbol P because those symbols have

TABLE 1–1

NAMES AND SYMBOLS OF ELEMENTS COMMONLY FOUND IN ORGANISMS

Name	Symbol
Calcium	Ca
Carbon	C
Chlorine	Cl
Copper	Cu
Hydrogen	H
Iodine	I
Iron	Fe
Magnesium	Mg
Nitrogen	N
Oxygen	O
Phosphorus	P
Potassium	K
Sodium	Na
Sulfur	S

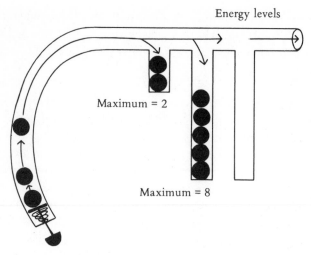

FIGURE 1-6
FILLING OF ENERGY LEVELS

already been assigned as described above. Instead sodium uses the name natrium for the symbol Na (remember, N is nitrogen) and potassium uses the name kalium for its symbol K.

The game we are playing has 106 kinds of players on the roster with each player wearing its own kind of jersey. The jersey lists the atomic symbol (naming the element), the atomic number (giving the number of protons or the number of electrons), and the atomic weight (usually permitting calculation of neutron number). In short, the basic structure of each atom is described.

ATOMS TO COMPOUNDS

The object of the game is to combine the atomic players into new molecules, new kinds of matter, that are needed by living systems. It is not possible to make all combinations of atoms. Only certain combinations are possible and these are determined by the rules of play. It is the outer portions of the atoms that meet and interact, namely the electrons. It is, therefore, the placement of the electrons within energy levels that determines how atoms interact, and this determines the rules of play.

ELECTRON PLACEMENT In all atoms, electrons are first placed in the lowest energy level nearest the nucleus (see Figure 1–6). This level can hold no more than two electrons, so the third electron, if present, must enter the second energy level. The second energy level can hold only eight electrons, the third through the tenth electrons for the atom. Therefore,

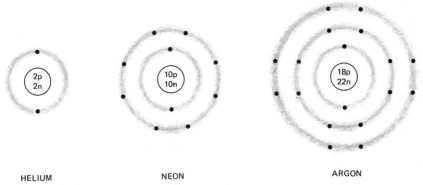

HELIUM   NEON   ARGON

FIGURE 1-7

**THE ATOMIC STRUCTURE OF HELIUM, NEON, AND
ARGON. IN EACH CASE THERE IS A FULL COMPLE-
MENT OF ELECTRONS IN THE OUTERMOST SHELL.
CONSEQUENTLY, THESE ELEMENTS DO NOT REACT
READILY WITH OTHER ELEMENTS. THEY ARE
CALLED INERT ELEMENTS. (P=PROTONS; N=NEUTRONS).**
Dickerson, Gray, and Haight, *Chemical Principles*, W. A. Benjamin, p. 295.

the eleventh electron, if present, must enter the third energy level. The
next seven electrons enter the third energy level, then the next two enter
the fourth energy level. After the twentieth electron, however, electron
placement follows a more complicated, but still definite pattern. For con-
venience sake, we will discuss only elements of atomic numbers one through
twenty. For our purposes we will say that the first energy level is complete
with two electrons, and the second, third, and fourth energy levels are
complete with eight electrons. Note, however, that in this book we will
never place more than two electrons in the fourth energy level, for that
would surpass our twenty electron limit.

The completeness of the outer energy level of an atom is very significant, for it is this, more than anything else, that determines the rules by
which atoms interact. Not only is this because the outermost energy level
is the one contacting the other atoms, but also it is because the inner
energy levels are already complete. The object of the game is to interact
with other atoms in one of three ways so that every atom involved in the
interaction has a complete outer energy level. Each atom in an interaction
may (1) lose one or more electrons to, (2) gain one or more electrons
from, or (3) share electrons with another atom.

Some atoms already have a complete outer energy level. These atoms
are *inert* or *nonreactive,* that is, they will not make any combinations at
all (see Figure 1-7). Helium, with atomic number two, is one example of
an inert element, and neon, with atomic number ten, is another. Remember, neon's first two electrons are the first energy level, and the remaining
eight complete the second energy level.

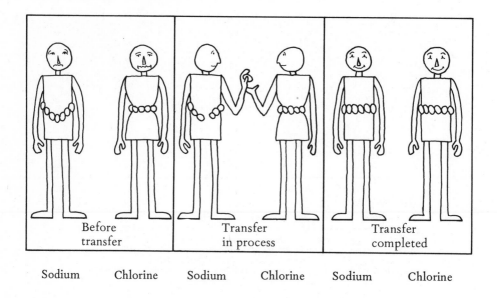

Before transfer		Transfer in process		Transfer completed	
Sodium	Chlorine	Sodium	Chlorine	Sodium	Chlorine

FIGURE 1-8

TRANSFER OF ELECTRONS Other atoms are very close to having a complete outer energy level, with either one electron too few or one or two too many (see Figure 1-8). In this case, the atom with one too few electrons strongly seeks another electron. As you can see, chlorine's electron belt is too tight. If it can find an atom with a loosely bound electron, it will capture that electron and not return it to its original owner. Alternatively, an atom like sodium, with one extra electron in its outer shell, has that electron only loosely bound. If it could lose that extra electron the next complete energy level underneath would become the outermost level.

This is one reason table salt is so easily formed. Table salt is sodium chloride. Sodium, with atomic number 11, has one outer electron and chlorine, with atomic number 17, has seven outer electrons. After the two atoms interact, sodium has a stable number of electrons, 10, and chlorine also has a stable number, 18, so the rules of play have been followed.

SHARING OF ELECTRONS Still other atoms have an in-between number of electrons in their outermost energy level. Carbon with atomic number six and four outer electrons is a prime example. Carbon can reach a stable electron number either by gaining four electrons to total eight in the outer level, or by losing the extra four it has. Because of its middle position, carbon does not have a strong tendency to either gain or lose, so instead it "compromises" and shares pairs of electrons with other atoms, with each partner donating one electron to the pair. By sharing we mean

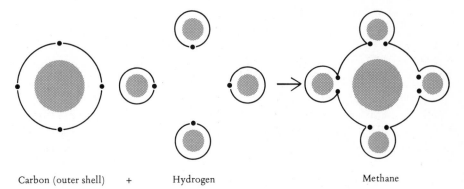

Carbon (outer shell)   +   Hydrogen   Methane

FIGURE 1–9

ELECTRON SHARING IS SHOWN SCHEMATICALLY. CARBON HAS FOUR ELECTRONS THAT IT MAY SHARE WITH OTHER ATOMS. EACH ATOM OF HYDROGEN HAS ONE ELECTRON TO SHARE. WHEN THE FOUR HYDROGEN ATOMS BOND TO THE CARBON ATOM, FOUR ELECTRON PAIRS FORM. THIS COMPLETES THE OUTER SHELL OF THE CARBON ATOM AND OF EACH HYDROGEN ATOM. Levy, *Elements of Biology*, 2/e. 1978. Addison-Wesley, Reading, MA. Fig. 2.8. Reprinted with permission.

that the electrons orbit first one atom, then the other, then return to the first. In other words, the electrons are not completely transferred.

But even if electrons are shared, they must still follow the rules of play. Every atom that enters the partnership must finish with at least a "share" of enough electrons to complete the outer energy level. Consider the natural gas methane as an example (see Figure 1–9). The carbon atom is interacting with four hydrogen atoms. Each hydrogen atom needs one more electron so each can put only one electron into a partnership in return for one of carbon's electrons to complete its outer level. Carbon, however, needs four electrons, not just one. Since each hydrogen can share only one electron, carbon combines with four different hydrogen atoms, gaining a share of one electron from each for a total of four. This completes carbon's outer level also and satisfies the rules of play.

IONIC AND COVALENT CHEMICAL BONDS When elements interact to form compounds, the atoms of each molecule are held together by a force called a *bond*. These bonds are created by the interaction of the electrons of the component atoms. Because there are two major kinds of electron interactions, there are also two kinds of bonds that form molecules. *Ionic bonds* are created when electrons are completely transferred from one atom to another. *Covalent bonds* are created when electrons are shared. Each type of bond exhibits different properties.

Ionic bonds result in the formation of *ions*, electrically charged atoms. Before two atoms interact each is electrically neutral with equal numbers of positive protons and negative electrons. When these same two atoms combine to form an ionicly bonded molecule, a negatively charged electron is transferred from one atom to the other, unbalancing both atoms. The atom losing the electron becomes a positively charged ion because one of its protons is no longer balanced by the lost electron. The other atom that gained a negatively charged electron becomes a negative ion. When the molecule is considered as a whole it is still neutral because the number of positive charges created equals the negative charges.

When an ionic bond is dissolved by water, it is possible to detect the presence of the charged ions. When in solution the positive and negative ions separate, but only slightly because of the attraction opposite charges have for each other. The close proximity and equal number of positive and negative charges prevent you from feeling these charges when you put your finger in such a solution. The charges can be detected, however, with the use of a battery and a meter that shows current flow. This is one reason an ionic solution is called an *electrolyte*—because it conducts electricity. Electrolytes are extremely important in biological systems because they permit proper nerve conduction, proper muscle contraction, and even proper function of all cell membranes.

In contrast to ionic bonds, covalent bonds do not dissociate in water and they do not conduct an electric current. They are *nonelectrolytes.* They usually form larger molecules than do ionic bonds and are more sturdy when dissolved in water, as all molecules in living systems are. For this reason, covalently bonded molecules form all major structures in living things.

Covalent bonds can exhibit some additional features. First, it is possible for the same two atoms to share more than one pair of electrons. When they share two pairs of electrons the bond between them is termed a *double bond,* and when they share three pairs of electrons it is called a *triple bond.* Multiple covalent bonds are found in common molecules such as carbon dioxide, shown in Figure 1–10.

Second, it is possible for two atoms to share a pair of electrons unequally. This occurs when the two atoms are unequal in their attraction of the electrons. Commonly this occurs when the atom with the larger, more positive nucleus possesses the shared pair a greater percentage of time. This creates a *polarity* of charges within a molecule because the atom having the electrons a greater percentage of time is slightly more negative than the other atom. The molecule is not ionic because the electrons are still shared; it is covalent but *polar.* Figure 1–11 shows a comparison of polar and nonpolar covalent molecules. Water is polar because oxygen has greater affinity for the shared electrons than hydrogen. Hydrogen gas, however, is nonpolar because the two hydrogen atoms have equal affinity for the electron pair so they share equally.

Single bond	H H | | H—C—C—H | | H H
Double bond	H H \ / C=C / \ H H
Triple bond	N≡N
Two double bonds	O=C=O

FIGURE 1-10

**REPRESENTATIVE COVALENT BOND. EACH HYDRO-
GEN ONLY MAKES ONE BOND, EACH OXYGEN
MAKES TWO BONDS, EACH NITROGEN MAKES
THREE BONDS, AND EACH CARBON MAKES FOUR
BONDS.**

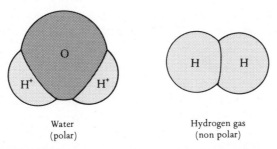

Water
(polar)

Hydrogen gas
(non polar)

FIGURE 1-11

**COMPARISON OF POLAR AND NONPOLAR COVALENT
MOLECULES, DENSITY INDICATES THE RELATIVE
DISTRIBUTION OF THE SHARED ELECTRONS.**

HYDROGEN BOND The polarity of hydrogen in many covalent molecules creates a form of bond called a *hydrogen bond.* A hydrogen bond is
much weaker than either an ionic or a·covalent bond, and unlike those two
bonds, it never occurs between adjacent atoms within one molecule but
rather holds together either different molecules or widely separated portions of the same molecule. A hydrogen bond occurs in extremely polar

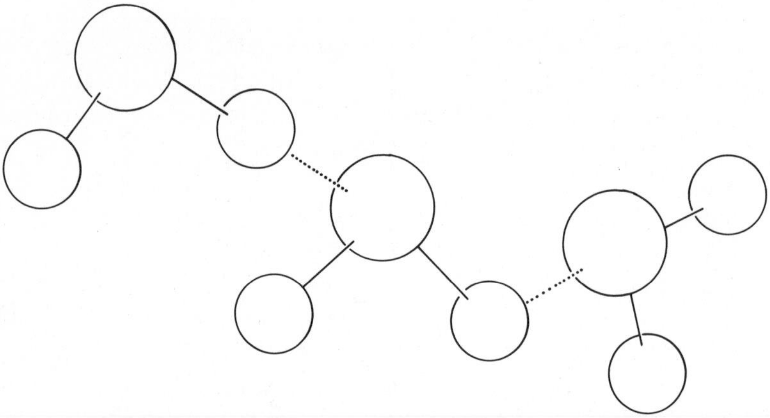

FIGURE 1-12

HYDROGEN BONDING IN WATER. THE HYDROGEN BONDS, REPRESENTED BY DOTS, ARE NOT AS STRONG AS COVALENT BONDS, BUT THEY DO CONTRIBUTE TO THE STABILITY OF STRUCTURES.

substances like water (see Figure 1–12) in which the nonhydrogen atom almost entirely monopolizes the electron pair leaving hydrogen positively charged. In such cases, the hydrogen is almost like a positive ion and it attracts the negative portion of another polar covalent molecule or of the same molecule. This attraction holds the two molecules or portions of a molecule together. As we shall see in later chapters, hydrogen bonding is very significant in living systems.

As we have seen, in all types of bonding, the significant factor is electron positioning. The type of bond formed depends greatly on the atoms interacting, the placement of their electrons in energy levels, the size of these atoms, and their overall attraction for electrons.

OXIDATION AND REDUCTION   The movement of electrons to or from each atom or group of atoms is so significant that there are special terms to describe it. *Reduction* is a gain of electrons and it results in a reduction of overall positive charge (due to negative charges acquired). Alternately, a loss of electrons is called *oxidation.* Perhaps this is because, more often than not the electrons lost by an atom go to oxygen. Since electrons do not just leave an atom without being attracted by another, oxidation (loss of electrons) never occurs without reduction (gain of electrons) occurring simultaneously to another atom. In fact, the atom or molecule reduced is called an *oxidizing agent* because it causes the oxidation of the other molecule. Similarly, the atom or molecule oxidized is called a *reducing agent* because it causes the reduction of the other molecule.

Oxidation and reduction, ionic and covalent bond formation, polarity and nonpolarity of molecules—these are all plays or moves in the game. The object of the game is to break bonds and make bonds, to gain, lose or share electrons from all possible sources in order to make the molecules needed by the storekeeper cell.

MOLECULAR FORMULAS The student of life functions is able to keep track of the play-by-play of the game by writing down all moves in a kind of chemical shorthand. The symbols used are the atomic symbols of the atom-players' names. All combinations made by the players are recorded in listings called *molecular formulas* that tell which atoms and how many of each combine. For example, the molecular formula of water is H_2O meaning two atoms of hydrogen and one of oxygen are combined. The formula for carbon dioxide is CO_2 meaning one atom of carbon and two of oxygen are combined. Table salt, sodium chloride, is written NaCl, meaning one atom of sodium and one of chlorine are combined. Remember, the lower case "a" and lower case "l" indicate that "Na" is one element and "Cl" is a second element.

STRUCTURAL FORMULAS Notice also that although the molecular formulas indicate the number and kinds of atoms combined they say nothing about placement. This information is obtainable only from *structural formulas* which are effective diagrams of atom placement within the molecules. Single bonds are indicated by one straight line between atoms, double bonds by two lines, and triple bonds by three lines. For example, the structural formula of water,

$$\begin{array}{c} O \\ / \quad \backslash \\ H \quad H \end{array}$$

indicates that the oxygen separates the two hydrogen atoms rather than them being in a series like this: H—H—O. Carbon dioxide's structural formula is O = C = O indicating that carbon shares two pairs of electrons (double bond) with each oxygen atom and that it is located between them. Unless atom position is important to a particular point being made, the molecular formula is more commonly used than the structural formula.

EQUATIONS DESCRIBE REACTIONS Now that we have a way of describing the player combinations made, all that is required is a simple way of describing the action. This is the function of the *equation*.

$$\underset{\text{reactant(s)}}{2\,H_2 + O_2} \xrightarrow[\text{catalyst(s)}]{\text{co-factor(s)}} \underset{\text{product(s)}}{2\,H_2O}$$

Beginning ingredients are called *reactants* and the molecules they rearrange to form are called *products*. The symbol for action is an arrow. By convention, reactants are usually written to the left of the arrow and the products they rearrange to form are on the right. Notice that the same players or atoms are in both reactants and products, they are merely rearranged.

At times, there are factors that affect the play, the combinations, without becoming part of them. These may be things like the starting gun or the coach's yelling. It's not really part of the action but it does alter the speed at which it occurs. These factors are written on the arrow and they include such things as *co-factors* and *catalysts*.

Catalysts are chemicals that increase the speed of a reaction without changing the end result. They cannot, therefore, become part of the products. As a result, they are released unchanged and may be reused. Co-factors are usually substances like vitamins that activate catalysts in living systems by becoming part of them. They too may be reused and, therefore, belong on the arrow of the equation.

Having discussed the components of a reaction we have completed our treatment of matter and some of its basic interactions. In the next chapter we will consider the role of hydrogen in living systems, another concept that is basic to the games cells play.

Chapter 2
MORE BASICS
Acids and Bases

Water composes over 90 percent of all living things. For this reason, most of the chemicals composing living things are in solution (dissolved). Not only must each chemical obey the general rules of play that we studied in Chapter 1, but also each chemical must behave in water in a characteristic manner. Substances called *acids* and *bases (alkalis)* are among the kinds of chemicals affected by water because water has components that may be attracted by both kinds of substances (see Figure 2–1).

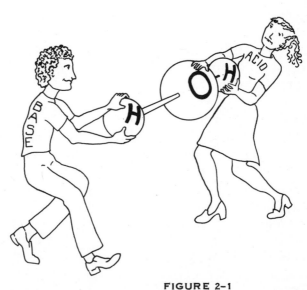

FIGURE 2–1
ACID–BASE TUG O'WAR

THE SIGNIFICANCE OF ACIDS AND BASES   Acids and bases are significant chemicals in living systems for two major reasons. First, both acids and bases are commonly found in living systems. Many waste products produced by cells in the game of survival are acidic or basic. Even water itself has acidic and basic components. A second reason that acids and bases are significant in living systems is that they may potentially harm those systems. Both kinds of chemicals readily react with the larger molecules that compose the structure of living systems and with the chemical catalysts that control the rate of reactions throughout the living system. The interaction of acids and bases with these chemicals changes their structure so they are no longer able to function properly and the living system is damaged both structurally and functionally. Therefore, organisms must regulate the acids and bases within them if they are to survive because of both the availability of these substances and the potential harm they can cause the organism.

DEFINITIONS   Acids and bases are described in many ways including their observable properties, their behavior in water, and their ability to donate or accept protons. Acidic properties include a sour taste in water (lemons contain acid) and the ability to turn litmus dye to pink. On the other hand, alkaline or basic properties include a bitter taste in water, a characteristic slippery feel, and the ability to turn litmus dye to blue.

Acids are defined as those substances that increase the *hydrogen ion* (H^+) concentration in water. Bases are defined as those substances which increase the *hydroxyl ion* (OH^-) concentration in water. These acids and bases may not contain a hydrogen ion or hydroxyl ion themselves but rather they may react with components of water to produce a predominance of one or the other ion. Before the interaction, water has equal concentrations of hydrogen and hydroxyl ions. Acids and bases react with water to change this balance (Figure 2–2).

EXAMPLES   Ammonia (NH_3) is an example of a base because it can combine with a hydrogen ion from water to form an ammonium ion (NH_4^+). This hydrogen ion is thus no longer balancing the effects of a hydroxyl ion, so the result is a solution with more hydroxyl ions than hydrogen ions. Ammonia, therefore, is a base because when it's placed in water it results in the production of excess hydroxyl ions.

On the other hand, carbon dioxide is an example of a gas that produces hydrogen ions when placed in solution. Carbon dioxide (CO_2) combines with water (H_2O) to produce carbonic acid (H_2CO_3). The carbonic acid, in turn, dissociates to form hydrogen ion (H^+) and bicarbonate ion (HCO_3^-). Therefore, it is possible for substances placed in water to create a predominance of either hydroxyl ions (as does ammonia) or hydrogen

A. Ammonia forms a base when it combines with water.

$$NH_3 + H^+ + OH^- \longrightarrow NH_4^+ + OH^-$$

ammonia water   ammonium   hydroxyl
                                ion   ion (no longer balanced
                                             by H^+)

B. Carbon dioxide forms an acid when it combines with water.

$$CO_2 + H_2O^- \longrightarrow H_2CO_3 \longrightarrow H^+ + HCO_3^-$$

Carbon water   carbonic   hydrogen ion   bicarbonate
dioxide   acid   (no longer   ion
                                            balanced by
                                           OH^-)

FIGURE 2–2

THE FORMATION OF BASES AND ACIDS IN SOLUTION

ions (as does carbon dioxide) even though these ions are not part of the original molecule. Production of these ions occurs due to an interaction with the water molecules.

The components of water can themselves be considered as acidic and basic. Although water is a covalent molecule it does ionize to a small but consistent degree. Specifically, water is .0000002 percent dissociated, or, stated another way, one molecule in 500 million is ionized into one hydrogen ion and one hydroxyl ion. Because pure water has equal numbers of acidic and alkaline components that cancel each other's effect, when considered as a whole water is neutral, neither acidic nor alkaline.

THE RELATIONSHIP OF H^+ AND OH^- There is a predictable, constant relationship between the concentration of hydrogen ions and hydroxyl ions in all water-based solutions. The concentration of these two ions multiplied together always results in the same number, called water's ionization constant. This relationship implies that if either ion increases in concentration, the other has to decrease in order to have their product still equal the constant. Thus the more hydrogen ions there are present in a solution, the fewer hydroxyl ions are present and vice versa.

THE pH SCALE To more clearly illustrate the relationship of hydrogen ions and hydroxyl ions, scientists derived a mathematically based scale called a pH *scale* (see Figure 2–3). The scale ranges from zero to fourteen, a number based upon the water constant previously described. The total of the hydrogen ion representation on the scale plus the hydroxyl ion on the scale is always equal to fourteen. Thus, if hydrogen accounts for four points on the scale, hydroxyl fills the remaining ten points. If hydrogen

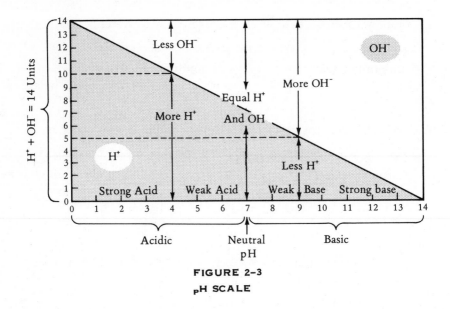

FIGURE 2–3

pH SCALE

TABLE 2–1

SOME MEASURED pH VALUES

Material	pH
1-molar HCl Solution	0.0
Gastric juice	1.4
Lemon juice	2.1
Orange juice	2.8
Sour pickles	3.0
Wine	3.5
Tomato juice	4.1
Black coffee	5.0
Peas	6.0
Rainwater	6.5
Milk	6.9
Pure water at 24°C	7.0
Blood	7.4
Baking soda solution	8.5
Borax solution	9.2
Limewater	10.5
Household ammonia	11.9
1-molar NaOH solution	14.0

is nine points on the scale, then hydroxyl is five points. If only the hydrogen ion value is stated, the hydroxyl ion value can automatically be determined by subtracting hydrogen's number from fourteen. Therefore both acidic solutions (with more hydrogen than hydroxyl ions) and basic solutions (with more hydroxyl than hydrogen ions) may be described in terms of the amount of hydrogen ion present, that is, their pH. Table 2–1 shows some common solutions and their approximate pH's.

The pH scale has the advantage of dealing in simple numbers between zero and fourteen rather than in complicated concentrations of hydrogen ion. The scale is extremely handy to use once the significance of each position is understood. The pH of seven is neutral, because it is there that hydrogen ions (seven on the scale) and hydroxyl ions (the remaining seven on the scale to total fourteen) are equal in concentration. Numbers below seven represent acids and numbers above seven represent bases. The farther away from seven the pH is, the stronger is the acid or base. For example, both pH one and pH six are acids because they are both below pH seven, but pH one is more acid than pH six because it is farther away from neutral seven. Similarly, both pH eight and pH thirteen are basic because they are both above pH seven, but pH thirteen is more basic because it is farther away from neutral seven.*

STRONG AND WEAK ACIDS AND BASES Of the many different chemicals that combine with water to form acidic and basic solutions, some are *weak acids or bases* (producing pH's nearer to seven) and others are *strong acids or bases* (producing pH's farther away from seven). This may be true even though identical amounts of the original chemicals were placed in equal volumes of water. This phenomenon can be best explained in terms of the tendency for each chemical, whether acid or base, to ionize when placed in water (see Figure 2–4).

Strong acids and bases may be likened to a party prankster's jar of "peanuts" that really contains coiled snakes mounted on strong springs. When a guest opens the jar, the snakes fly out. In a similar manner, hydrogen ions or hydroxyl ions seem to "fly out" of a strong chemical when it is placed in water (the jar is opened). A weak acid or base is like the same prank item mounted with weak springs. The same number of snakes (hydrogen and hydroxyl ions) are potentially present, but they never get out of the jar *(dissociate).*

---

*Although this concept of the interpretation of the pH scale is very simple, many beginning students find it confusing because low pH numbers mean high hydrogen ion concentrations. This is because the pH number represents the number of decimal places in a very small number. For example, the pH one represents the hydrogen ion concentration 0.1 (one decimal place) while pH six represents the hydrogen ion concentration 0.000001 (six decimal places). Because 0.1 (one tenth) is a much larger number than 0.000001 (one millionth), the pH one represents more hydrogen ions than pH six. Therefore, the lower the pH, the more hydrogen ions are present, and the more acidic is the solution.

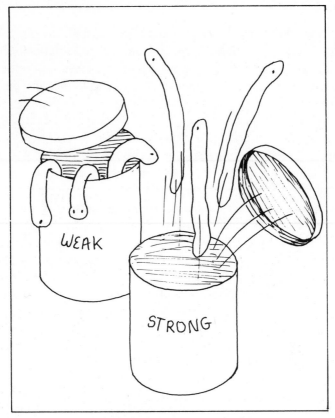

FIGURE 2–4
WEAK VS. STRONG ACIDS

The acidity or alkalinity of a solution is determined by free hydrogen and free hydroxyl ions. Those atoms that remain covalently bonded do not contribute to pH changes. As a result, acids like hydrogen chloride (HCl), with "strong springs" that ionize completely, form a lot of free hydrogen ions and are, therefore, strong acids. However, acids like carbonic acid (H_2CO_3) with "weak springs" only partially ionize to H^+ and HCO_3^- (bicarbonate ion), and are considered weak acids. Most of the acid remains together as H_2CO_3, does not form free hydrogen ions, and therefore, does not contribute to extreme pH change (see Figure 2–5).

Similarly there are strong and weak bases. Sodium hydroxide (NaOH) tends to ionize completely in water creating an abundance of hydroxyl ions and an extremely alkaline pH. Sodium hydroxide is, therefore, a strong base. On the other hand, ammonium hydroxide (NH_4OH) has less tendency to ionize, so for the same amount of chemical, less free OH^- is released. Therefore, ammonium hydroxide is a weaker base.

Interestingly, the strongness or weakness of an acid does not alter its ability to neutralize a base or vice versa. Whether strong or weak the same

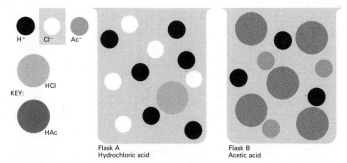

Flask A
Hydrochloric acid

Flask B
Acetic acid

FIGURE 2-5

WATER AND THE STRENGTH OF ACIDS AND BASES. DIAGRAMMATIC REPRESENTATION OF THE NUMBER OF HYDROGEN IONS PRESENT IN A SOLUTION OF STRONG ACID (SUCH AS HYDROCHLORIC) AND A SOLUTION OF WEAK ACID (SUCH AS CARBONIC). BECAUSE HYDROCHLORIC ACID IONIZES ALMOST 100 PERCENT, SOLUTIONS OF THIS ACID CONTAIN MANY FREE HYDROGEN IONS. CARBONIC ACID IONIZES ONLY ABOUT 1 PERCENT. AS A RESULT, SOLUTIONS OF THIS ACID CONTAIN FAR FEWER FREE HYDROGEN IONS. Baker and Allen, *Matter, Energy and Life*, 3rd edition, p. 95.

total number of hydrogen or hydroxyl ions are potentially available. As the few free hydrogen ions of a weak acid combine with the free hydroxyl of a base to form neutral water, more of the weak acid ionizes, creating more hydrogen ions that can neutralize more hydroxyl. The stepwise ionization occurs until the base is completely neutralized or the acid is completely used up.

SALTS The neutralization products that remain after an acid and base combine are called *salts*. For example, when the acid HCl exactly neutralizes the base NaOH, the H^+ and OH^- combine to form water. This leaves only Na^+ and Cl^- or common table salt (NaCl) in the water solution. If the acid H_2CO_3 neutralizes the base NaOH, the results are again water and a salt. This time, however, the salt is $NaHCO_3$ or sodium bicarbonate (baking soda).

The presence of weak acids, weak bases, and salts of these acids and bases in living systems is vital to survival because this combination is able to help stabilize pH. Each living system is able to survive only within a pH range specific to that organism. The human organism, for example, is able to *survive* only if its blood pH is between 6.9 and 7.9. It is *healthy* only if its blood pH is 7.33 to 7.45.* This is an extremely narrow range of pH

---

*Other specialized body fluids have different pH's. For example, gastric juice (from the stomach) has a pH of 1.4. This extreme pH is possible because a layer of mucus keeps this acidic fluid away from the stomach wall, preventing it from being absorbed into the blood stream and preventing it from damaging the stomach wall.

tolerance for an organism that is constantly producing acids and bases within its body. Without the presence of chemical systems capable of stabilizing pH, survival of such an organism would be tenuous at best. These pH stabilizers are called *buffers* and all living things possess them.

BUFFERS A buffer may be defined as a chemical or system of chemicals capable of combining with both free hydrogen ions and free hydroxyl ions to minimize all pH changes. In a way, a buffer is similar to a semimoistened sponge that mops up hydrogen ions instead of water (see Figure 2–6). The same sponge can perform two opposite functions. Because it is not yet saturated it may be used to mop up even more hydrogen ions when an excess is produced by the organism. Or the sponge may be wrung out to release the hydrogen ions it already contains, if these ions are needed to neutralize or combine with excess hydroxyl ions being produced by the organism. Like the sponge, a buffer is able to mop up or combine with excess hydrogen ions as well as excess hydroxyl ions. A buffer cannot stop pH change, it can only minimize it. This means that if a strong acid is added to a buffer solution, the pH will drop less than if the same acid were added to a nonbuffered solution. Likewise if a strong base were added to this same buffered solution the pH would increase less than if the same amount of base were added to a nonbuffered solution. The pH change is, therefore, minimized by the buffer but not prevented by it.

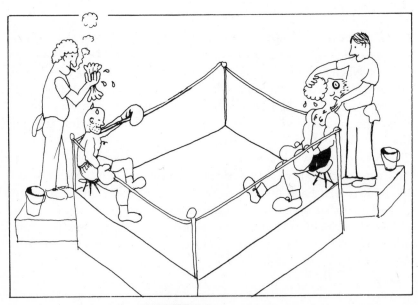

FIGURE 2–6
SPONGE AS A BUFFER

Most chemical buffer systems are composed of a weak acid or base and its salt. *Weak* acids or bases are required because the object is to keep the H^+ and OH^- *combined* and not freely ionized. The need for a salt of the acid or base can perhaps best be explained by example.

In most living systems an important buffer system is that of carbonic acid (H_2CO_3) and its salt, sodium bicarbonate ($NaHCO_3$) (Figure 2–7). Because carbonic acid is weak it does not drastically change the pH away from seven, yet it contains hydrogen ion (H^+) that is capable of neutralizing any free hydroxyl ion (OH^-) that may happen to enter the system. Thus, the carbonic acid portion of this buffer system is capable of minimizing the effects of a base added to the solution. The presence of the salt, sodium bicarbonate, is necessary to meet the second half of the requirements of a buffer system, the ability to combine with an acid to minimize its effects also. Hydrogen (H^+) ion combines with the bicarbonate ion (HCO_3^-) of the salt to produce weak carbonic acid (H_2CO_3). Because it is weak (or chiefly nonionized) very little of the hydrogen ion remains free and the pH changes relatively little. Thus, carbonic acid and sodium bicarbonate form a buffer system capable of minimizing pH changes in both the acid direction and the base direction.

Sometimes a buffer is composed of only one kind of molecule rather than a system of chemicals. Large proteins such as those contained in the molecule hemoglobin (Hb) are an example. The protein portion of hemoglobin is capable of combining with hydrogen ion to form what is called hydrogenated hemoglobin (HHb). At normal body pH only a portion of the hemoglobin molecules are hydrogenated (like the semimoistened sponge), so both Hb and HHb are present. If an excess of H^+ is produced it can attach to Hb to form more HHb and the change in pH is minimized.

Acid + Buffer System

$\boxed{H^+}$ + $\fbox{$H_2CO_3$ + Na + $\boxed{HCO_3^-}$}$ $\longrightarrow$ Forms more H_2CO_3

Base + Buffer System

$\boxed{OH^-}$ + $\fbox{$\boxed{H_2CO_3}$ + Na^+ + HCO_3^-}$ $\longrightarrow$ Forms H_2O + more HCO_3^-

FIGURE 2–7

THE CARBONIC ACID BUFFER SYSTEM. FREE H^+ AND FREE OH^- COMBINE WITH DIFFERENT COMPONENTS FO THE BUFFER SYSTEM. IN NEITHER CASE IS THE FREE H^+ OR FREE OH^- CONCENTRATION DRASTICALLY REDUCED.

Or, if an excess of OH⁻ is produced, H^+ can be released from HHb to neutralize the excess, forming harmless water and Hb. Again, the change in pH is minimized. Thus, hemoglobin (Hb and HHb) is an example of a buffer.

Because hydrogen ions and hydroxyl ions react readily with chemicals that compose living systems (such as proteins, fats, and carbohydrates) they can potentially change these chemicals and can cause severe damage to living organisms. It is this potential for harm as well as the ready availability of these ions to living systems that makes the presence of effective buffers vital to an organism's survival.

In the remaining chapters we will study the game in more detail. We will begin in the next section with a study of the principal players.

Self-Test

CHAPTER 1 THE BASICS

1. Write a definition for each of the following terms:
   a. atom:

   b. element:

   c. molecule:

   d. compound:

2. Describe the basic structure that is common to all atoms.

3. Which of the following subatomic particles determines the kind of element an atom is?
   a. proton
   b. neutron
   c. electron

4. Two electrically neutral atoms of the same element may have different numbers of:
   a. protons
   b. neutrons
   c. electrons

5. Match the description on the left with the term on the right. (answers may be used more than once)

    _____ 1. creates electrolytes

    _____ 2. shares two electrons (one pair) either equally or unequally

    _____ 3. electrons unequally shared

    _____ 4. results in ions

    _____ 5. loosely binds different molecules together

    a. hydrogen bond
    b. ionic bond
    c. double bond
    d. covalent bond
    e. polar molecule

6. The term _____ means a gain of electrons, while the term _____ is a loss of electrons.

7. Which of the following diagrams the position of the atoms in a molecule?
    a. molecular formula
    b. structural formula

8. In an equation, _____ are usually written on top of the arrow.
    a. catalysts
    b. products
    c. reactants

CHAPTER 2 MORE BASICS

1. Name two reasons acids and bases must be regulated in living systems.
    a.

    b.

2. Define an acid.

3. Define a base.

4. When hydrogen ion concentration decreases in an aqueous solution, hydroxyl ion concentration _____.

5. Match:
_____ 1. a solution of pH 4   a. acidic
_____ 2. a solution of pH 6   b. alkaline
_____ 3. a solution of pH 8   c. neutral
_____ 4. a solution with more hydroxyl
        ion than hydrogen ion
_____ 5. a solution with more hydrogen
        ion than hydroxyl

6. Match the pH with the description.
_____ 1. pH 12   a. strong acid
_____ 2. pH 2   b. weak acid
_____ 3. pH 4   c. strong base
_____ 4. pH 8   d. weak base

7. A given amount of strong acid can neutralize more base than the same amount of a weak acid.
   a. true
   b. false

8. Define a buffer.

9. Which component of the bicarbonate buffer system is able to combine with hydrogen ion? _____
   with hydroxyl ion? _____

10. Name one buffer besides the bicarbonate buffer system that is found in many living systems (including the human).

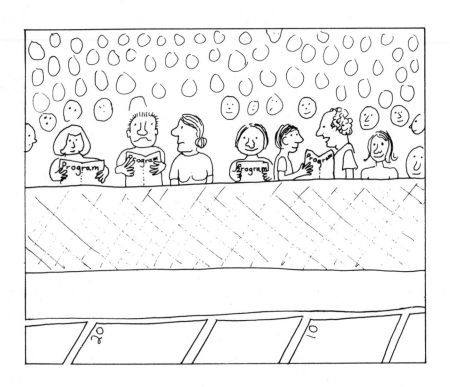

Section Two
The Players

OBJECTIVES FOR SECTION TWO

Chapter 3
ELEMENTS OF LIFE: Carbon, Hydrogen, Oxygen, Nitrogen, plus Water

1. Identify the three most abundant chemical elements found in living organisms.
2. Identify the properties of the element carbon which account for the stability and versatility of its compounds in living systems.
3. Identify the properties of the element oxygen which suit it for its role in the chemistry of life.
4. Describe the structure of the water molecule and relate the solvent and hydrogen bonding properties of water to this structure.

Chapter 4
MOLECULES OF LIFE: Protein, Carbohydrate, Lipid, and Nucleic Acids

1. Recognize a literal definition for carbohydrates and identify the importance of carbohydrates in the living world.
2. Define monosaccharide and classify selected monosaccharides according to the number of carbon atoms each contains.
3. Show an understanding of isomers by indicating why glucose and galactose are said to be isomers of one another.
4. State why maltose is an appropriate example of an oligosaccharide.
5. Define the process of dehydration synthesis.
6. Define polysaccharides and identify the functions of two selected polysaccharides: starch and cellulose.
7. Recognize a general definition of lipids.
8. Identify the components of a neutral fat and state why neutral fats play a prominent role in long term energy storage.
9. Recognize the structural features of phospholipids which make them well suited as building blocks of cell membranes.
10. Define proteins and list or recognize five functions which can be attributed to different types of proteins.
11. Describe the common structural features of all amino acids and indicate how the amino acids differ from one another.
12. Recognize descriptions of the four levels of organization found in protein molecules.
13. Identify the principle role of nucleic acids.
14. Identify the three components of a DNA (deoxyribonucleic acid) nucleotide, and recognize or state the base pairing rules for DNA.
15. List three features which distinguish RNA (ribonucleic acid) from DNA.

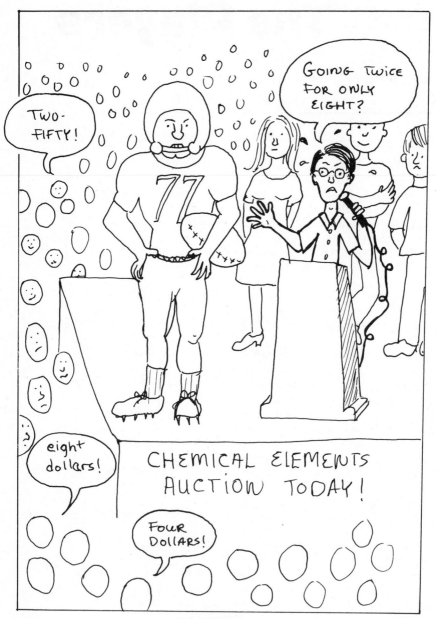

FIGURE 3-1
SOLD CHEAP!

Chapter 3
ELEMENTS OF LIFE
Carbon, Hydrogen, Oxygen, Nitrogen, plus Water

In both the literature and in conversations dealing with religion, philosophy, and politics there is often great debate over the worth of a human life, with one commonly held opinion being that a human is priceless. If, however, we were to "price" a human in terms of the chemical elements of which he or she is composed, we would find that there is very little debate about a human's value and, in fact, very little value. As our introductory cartoon (Figure 3-1) indicates, unless a person has gold fillings or a platinum heart valve, the sum total of all the chemical elements in a body are worth about ten dollars. Therefore, since the elements that make up the body have obviously not been selected for their dollar value, we might ask, "why have they been chosen?" We will focus on this question later in this chapter, but first let's consider just what these "cheap" elements of life are.

The left hand column of Table 3-1 lists the elements that are found in living organisms, along with their relative abundance in the middle column. A study of this table shows that without question the most abundant elements associated with life are hydrogen, carbon, and oxygen, since these three elements alone account for 99 percent of all the atoms in an organism. It might be tempting to suggest that these elements are most abundant in organisms because they are also most abundant in the earth's crust.

The right hand column of Table 3-1, however, shows that this is not true. Hydrogen, for instance, constitutes 49 percent of all of the atoms in an organism, while only comprising 0.22 per cent of the earth's crust. On the other hand, silicon makes up 49 per cent of the earth's crust, but it constitutes only 0.033 per cent of the atoms in an organism. If, therefore, the atoms commonly found in an organism were selected neither for their

(a)

(b)

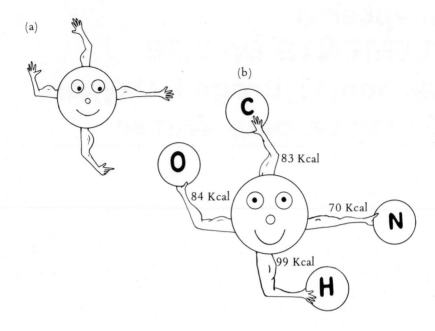

(c)

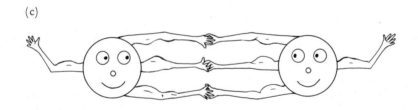

(d)

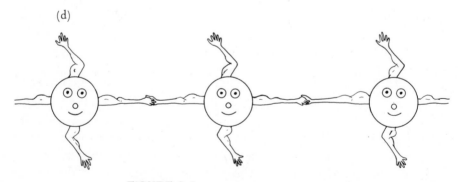

FIGURE 3-2
BONDING PROPERTIES OF CARBON

TABLE 3-1

RELATIVE PERCENTAGES OF ELEMENTS
FOUND IN LIVING ORGANISMS VS. THE
EARTH'S CRUST

Element	Organisms*	Earth's crust†
Hydrogen	49	0.22
Carbon	25	0.19
Oxygen	25	47
Nitrogen	0.27	<0.1
Calcium	0.073	3.5
Potassium	0.046	2.5
Silicon	0.033	28
Magnesium	0.031	2.2
Phosphorus	0.030	<0.1
Sodium	0.015	2.5
Others	Traces	13.7

*From E. S. Deevey, *Scientific American*, (September, 1970), p. 149
†From E. Frieden, *Scientific American*, (July, 1972), p. 52.

value nor for their abundance on the earth, they must have been chosen
for the possession of certain chemical properties which we will now
examine.

CARBON   The atom to be considered first is carbon. It serves as the key
atom in most of the molecules in an organism, and is so important that
some scientists state that the chemistry of life is really the chemistry of
carbon. What, then, is so special about carbon? For openers, it is a light
element with an atomic number of six. Having six protons, it also has six
electrons, with four of them being located in its outer shell. Because a
stable number of electrons for this shell is eight, carbon tends to achieve
stability by gaining a share in four more electrons through the formation
of four covalent bonds. This bonding tendency is represented in Figure
3-2 by the four arms attached to our imaginary carbon. Carbon can form
these bonds with a number of elements with differing chemical properties,
such as hydrogen, oxygen, nitrogen, and even other carbon atoms. Figure
3-2b shows carbon achieving a stable state by forming a covalent bond
with each of the atoms mentioned above. This part of the figure, however,
further emphasizes an important point, namely that the covalent bonds
that involve carbon are extremely strong bonds requiring much energy to
break. The numbers along each muscular arm stand for the amount of

energy in kilocalories (Kcal) needed to break each specific bond. Because they are so high, carbon would make an ideal catcher in a chemical trapeze act. When carbon, for example, is covalently bonded to another carbon, the bond would not be broken until 83 Kcal of energy were supplied. That such a bond is a strong bond can be seen by comparing the amount of energy needed to break a Si–Si bond. In this case the energy required is only about one-half that needed to break a C–C bond, namely 42 Kcal. Silicon, therefore, although it is related to carbon, would be a poor choice for the job of catcher in the trapeze act. Because of the relative weakness of its bonds, silicon compounds tend to be unstable, while the compounds containing the strong-bonding carbon are very stable. This property of forming stable compounds, therefore, is one reason why carbon is the key element in the highly organized and relatively stable system we call an organism.

Parts c and d of Figure 3–2, provide additional information relative to carbon's important role in the chemistry of life. In Part c of the figure we see that carbon can fulfill its need to gain a share in four additional electrons by forming multiple bonds, that is, by sharing more than one electron pair with the same atom. In practice, double or triple bonds are possible when either two or three pairs of electrons respectively are shared between carbon and another atom. In our figure "Mr. Carbon" is engaged in a triple bond with three pairs of electrons being shared with another carbon atom.

Finally, Part d of Figure 3–2 points out still another feature, which follows from carbon's tendency to form four covalent bonds. In this case, we show a number of carbon atoms linked together to form a long chain of carbons, which can serve as the backbone for many different compounds. Moreover, just as it is possible to arrange a number of similar beads into a variety of different pieces of jewelery by forming branching networks and rings, so too carbon atoms can be joined together in a variety of ways to form different compounds. Carbon, therefore, is well-suited for the chemistry of life not only because of the stability of the compounds in which it is found, but also because of its versatility, that is, its ability to be the central atom in a virtually endless number of different compounds.

OXYGEN A second element essential to living organisms is oxygen. One property of oxygen that makes it important for life is its ability to serve as a sort of taxi for the transportation of carbon from organism to organism (see Figure 3–3). When carbon combines with a molecule of oxygen (O_2), the stable gas carbon dioxide is formed. Moreover, this gas, as well as oxygen itself, is soluble in water thereby assuring its ability to reach water-

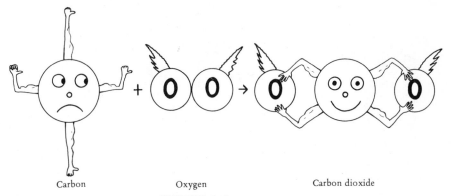

Carbon   Oxygen   Carbon dioxide

FIGURE 3–3
CARBON TRANSPORT

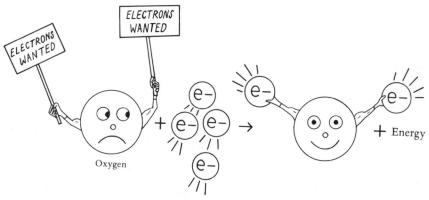

Oxygen

FIGURE 3–4
OXYGEN AS AN ELECTRON ACCEPTOR

dwelling as well as land-dwelling organisms. In addition, because it is a small element (atomic number 8) needing to gain only two electrons to achieve a stable state, oxygen is a strong electron seeker. This means, as Figure 3–4 demonstrates, that frequently energy is given off when electrons are transferred to oxygen. Such a transfer is at the roots of an extremely important energy yielding process in living organisms known as *respiration*—a process we'll consider at length in a later chapter of this book.

HYDROGEN AND WATER Up to this point we have considered the importance of the elements carbon and oxygen. The third and most abundant element in organisms is hydrogen. One reason for its abundance is that hydrogen readily forms covalent bonds with carbon atoms. Hydrogen, however, also readily bonds with oxygen to form the familiar compound

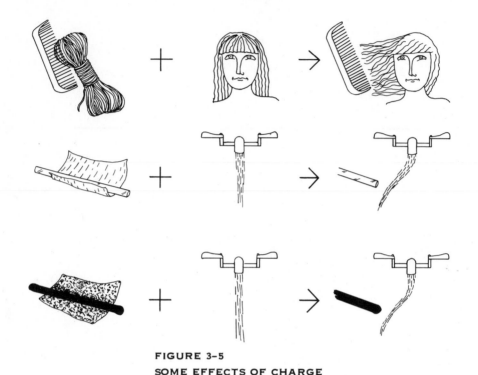

FIGURE 3-5
SOME EFFECTS OF CHARGE

water, H_2O. When one realizes that living cells consist of from 60 to 95 per cent water, its importance to life seems obvious. But why has life evolved with such a dependence on this apparently simple compound? The answer stems largely from the structure of the water molecule.

Part a of Figure 3-5 demonstrates a phenomenon which you might already have experienced or which you might like to try. If a comb is rubbed with a piece of wool cloth and then brought near a person's head, the hair on the head is attracted to the comb and appears to stand on end. The explanation of this phenomenon is that a charge was induced on the comb by rubbing it with the wool. Apparently then, the charged comb attracted opposite charges in the hair drawing it toward the comb, just as the opposing poles of two magnets are drawn together. At this point you are probably saying, "that's nice but what does it have to do with water?" Part b of Figure 3-5 helps to explain. Here a glass rod is rubbed with a piece of silk to induce a positive charge on it. If this charged rod is then brought close to a stream of water, the stream bends toward it. Since this situation is similar to that of the comb and the hair, the explanation of this phenomenon must be similar, namely that the stream of water bends

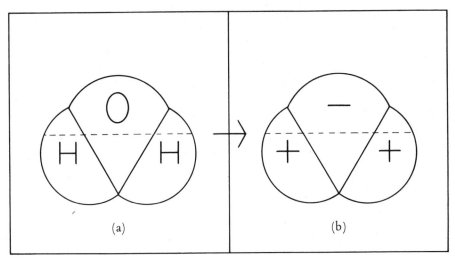

FIGURE 3-6
STRUCTURE OF THE WATER MOLECULE

because its molecules exhibit an opposite or negative charge. Moreover, the experiment can be repeated using a rubber rod charged with a piece of wool. In this case the charge on the rod is negative. When it is brought toward a stream of water, however, the water again bends toward the rod, indicating that the water molecules exhibit a positive charge as well as the negative charge demonstrated above.

How can these observations be related to the structure of the water molecule? In Figure 3-6a you see a space-filling model of one such molecule.

Notice that the molecule is not linear, that is, the two hydrogen atoms are not in a straight line with the oxygen atom, but rather they are off to one side or below the imaginary line drawn through the molecule. What consequences does this lack of symmetry have? Well, recall earlier that one property of oxygen that was mentioned was its tendency to attract or seek electrons. Since oxygen has this great attraction for electrons, the electrons shared between the hydrogen and oxygen spend more time at the oxygen end of the molecule rather than at the hydrogen end. The consequences are shown in Figure 3-6b, namely that the oxygen end of the molecule exhibits a negative charge (attraction to the positively charged glass rod) and the hydrogen end exhibits a positive charge (attraction to the negatively charged rubber rod), that is, the molecule is polar.

What then are some of the useful properties of water that depend upon its structure? One function of water in the cells of an organism is to act as a *solvent*. In fact, water is such a good solvent in the living system

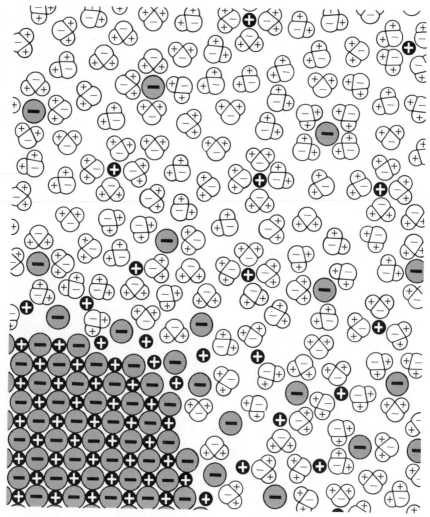

FIGURE 3–7
WATER ACTING AS A SOLVENT

that it is sometimes referred to as the universal solvent of life. Figure 3–7 shows how water is effective as a dissolving agent, or solvent, for an ionic or charged substance like salt. Notice in the figure that the oppositely charged ends of the water molecules surround each appropriate ion. Moreover, water is also able to *dissolve* a large number of *organic molecules,* * which exhibit a partial separation of charge in pretty much the same fashion.

---

*Nearly all carbon-containing compounds.

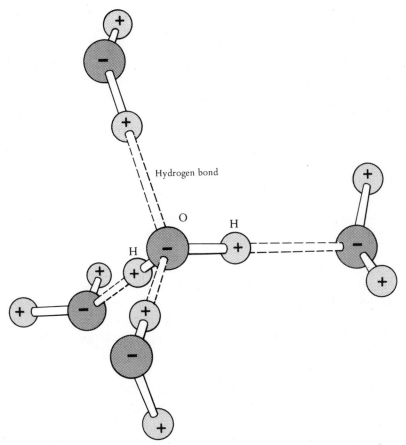

Hydrogen bond

O

H

H

FIGURE 3-8
HYDROGEN BONDING BETWEEN WATER MOLECULES

HYDROGEN BONDS Water molecules, however, are not attracted only to ions or other charged molecules: by virtue of their own oppositely charged ends, they are also attracted to one another. Such attractions, shown by the dashed lines in Figure 3-8, are strong enough to create bonds between adjacent water molecules. These are known as hydrogen bonds. In ice all of the water molecules are involved in hydrogen bonds to form a rigid lattice. When ice melts, however, water molecules can move closer together. Ice, therefore, is less dense than liquid water, and as a result forms at the surface of a body of water. If you were a fish, this would be important to you because this is why a body of water freezes from the top down rather than in the reverse direction.

The hydrogen bonding properties of water, however, are important to you and me at higher temperatures. All liquids can be converted to a gas provided enough energy is available for the individual molecules to escape from the surface of the liquid. The molecules of some substances that show very little attraction for one another require relatively little energy to escape into the gaseous state. An example you're probably familiar with is swabbing your forehead with alcohol when you have a fever. The alcohol readily evaporates, and you feel cooler because the heat energy present in your forehead is used to vaporize the alcohol. Water, unlike alcohol, doesn't vaporize as readily. Applied to your forehead, most of it would just roll off as a liquid. Why? The explanation is that the hydrogen bonds *between* water molecules have to be broken before an individual molecule can escape into the gaseous state. In other words, more energy must be supplied to free individual water molecules. The implication for us, therefore, is that we can dissipate a large amount of body heat by evaporating only a small amount of water from our body fluids.

In this chapter, we have considered some of the chemical properties of the three most abundant elements of life: carbon, oxygen, and hydrogen. Of course, as Table 3-1 indicates, other elements are found in lesser amounts in living organisms, and we will consider the unique roles of some of these elements in subsequent chapters. We have implied, however, that the atoms of elements do not exist in organisms in isolation. More frequently, they are found as components of certain special types of large molecules such as carbohydrates and proteins. In our next chapter then, we will consider the major groups of the molecules of life.

Chapter 4
MOLECULES OF LIFE
Protein, Carbohydrate, Lipid, and Nucleic Acids

In the last chapter we made a big point about humans and, for that matter, all organisms, being relatively worthless or at best inexpensive when considered at the level of the chemical elements of which they are composed. If, however, we consider the more complex level of the molecules in which these elements are utilized, a human can truly be considered a "six-million-dollar man." This enormous price tag stems from the fact that the living organism can manufacture many molecules that are such architectural marvels that the scientist, with the benefit of all of his or her wisdom and technical wizardry, isn't even able to approach them.

These most complex molecular players of life are organic molecules known as *proteins* and *nucleic acids.* They have as team mates, however, two other classes of molecules, the *carbohydrates* and *lipids,* so in this chapter we will consider the chemical natures and functions of each of these team members.

CARBOHYDRATES The players who literally provide the spark or energy for the rest of the team are the carbohydrates. The name translates as "carbon held by water" and is derived from the general formula for this group of molecules, which is $C_n(H_2O)_n$, where n stands for the number of carbon atoms in the molecule. This formula says, therefore, that for every carbon atom present, the elements of water, namely two hydrogen atoms and an oxygen atom, are also present. Carbohydrates can be considered the team spark plug, because their principal role is energy conversion. Just as a wood log is consumed in fire to provide energy in the forms of heat and light, certain carbohydrates are consumed in chemical reactions to provide chemical energy for all of the team's activities.

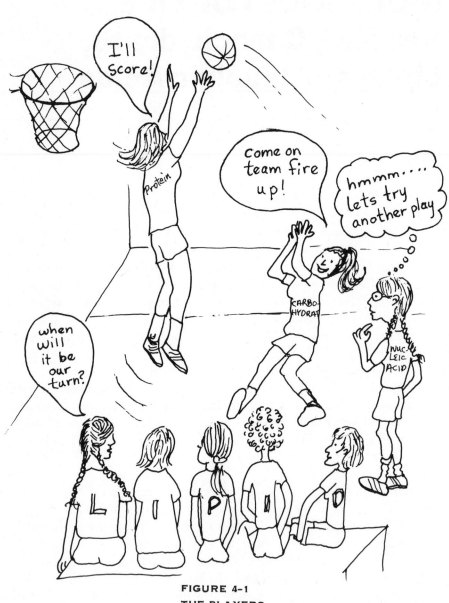

FIGURE 4-1
THE PLAYERS

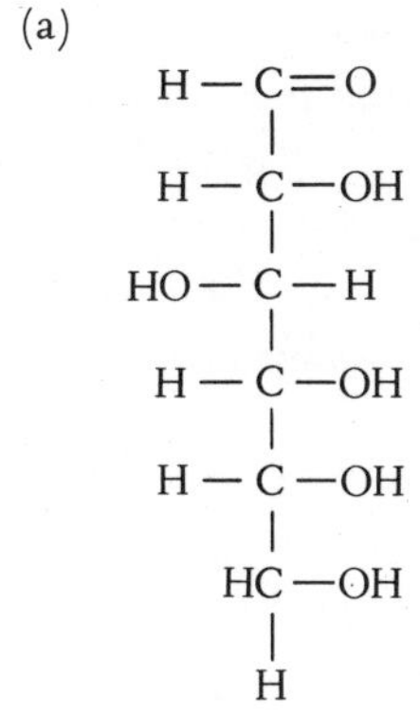

(a)

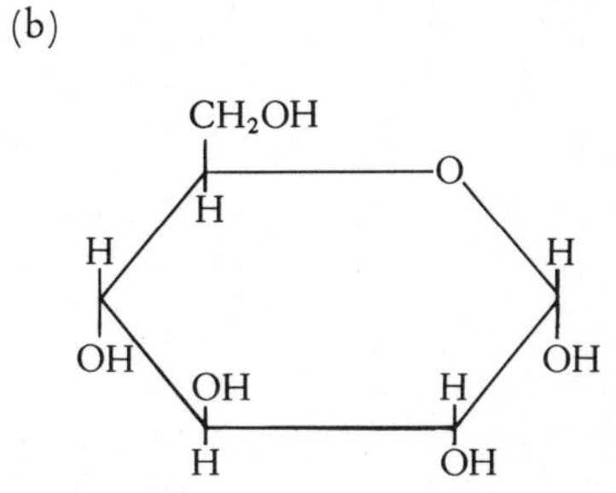

(b)

FIGURE 4-2

TWO REPRESENTATIONS OF THE CARBOHYDRATE, GLUCOSE

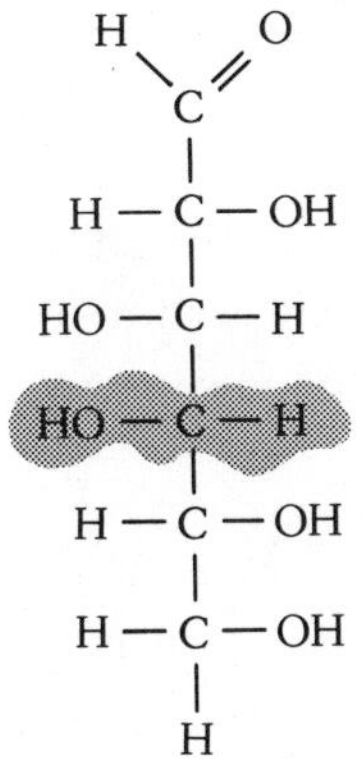

FIGURE 4-3

GALACTOSE, AN ISOMER OF GLUCOSE

The carbohydrate that directly sacrifices itself for the team in this way is *glucose.* It is composed of a *single* sugar unit, and as such is known as a *monosaccharide* (one sugar). Figure 4–2a shows one structural representation of this molecule.

Its carbon backbone should be quite evident from this figure, as should the hydrogen and hydroxyl groups "hydrating" the carbon. By counting atoms, you should convince yourself that glucose fits the general formula for carbohydrates, namely $C_n(H_2O)_n$. For glucose what does the n in this formula stand for? Part b of Figure 4–2 shows a second structural representation of the same glucose molecule. You should recall from the last chapter that the carbon backbone can form rings as well as chains. Figure 4–2b, therefore, shows the ring form of glucose. A count of the atoms in this figure should convince you that the ring form contains the same number of atoms as the so-called straight chain form of glucose. Be careful, however, not to conclude that all molecules having the same number of atoms are necessarily identical to one another. Consider the molecule in Figure 4–3.

You might be tempted to say that this is just a repeat of Figure 4–2a. There is, however, a difference as indicated by the shaded part of the figure. The hydrogen and hydroxyl group attached to this particular carbon atom have been shifted to opposite sides. Is this an important difference? Well, just as reversible skirts and vests allow one to give a different look to one's wardrobe without actually buying more clothes, so too the reversing or shifting of atoms in a molecule give that molecule a different look. The difference is sufficient enough, in fact, to warrant naming the sugar in Figure 4–3 galactose rather than glucose. Molecules such as glucose and galactose, which have the same molecular formula but a different structural arrangement of atoms, are said to be *isomers* of one another, and as you might imagine, the existence of isomers greatly increases the number of different compounds that can be found in an organism.

As I hope you determined for yourself a few minutes ago, glucose and galactose are monosaccharides that both contain six carbon atoms. They, therefore, belong to a group of monosaccharides known as *hexoses. Hex* is from the Greek meaning six and *ose* is a common ending for all sugars. Other monosaccharides containing differing numbers of carbon atoms are named in similar fashion, and some of this terminology is summarized in Table 4–1.

TABLE 4–1

Number of carbon atoms	Group name	Common examples
3	triose	glyceraldehyde
4	tetrose	erythrose
5	pentose	ribose, deoxyribose
6	hexose	glucose, galactose, fructose

In addition to a variety of monosaccharides, the carbohydrates are represented by a group of sugars known as *oligosaccharides.* Just as an oligarchy is a form of government in which supreme power is restricted to a *few,* so too an oligosaccharide is a carbohydrate composed of a *few* simple sugar units jointed together. (Actually the number of units can vary from two to nine.) One of the simplest oligosaccharides is the *disaccharide* maltose because it is composed of only two (di) identical glucose molecules. The formation of maltose is outlined in Figure 4–4.

As the figure indicates, the two glucose subunits in maltose are linked together by an oxygen bridge. Moreover, this bridge is formed at the expense of the removal of a water molecule. The formation of maltose in this manner is an example of a reaction known as a *dehydration synthesis.* Dehydration means loss of water, whether it be from a person sweating in

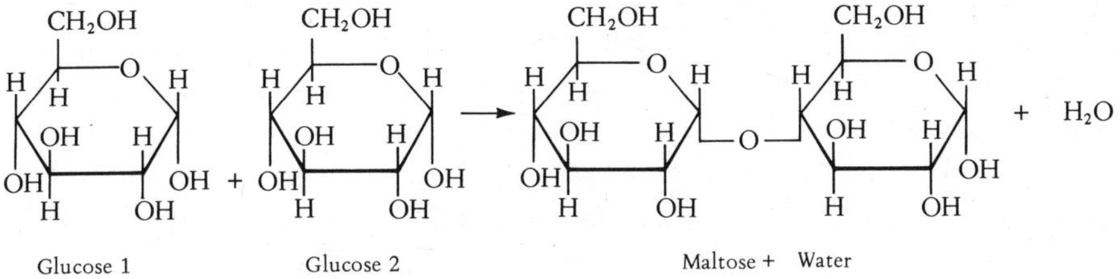

Glucose 1   Glucose 2   Maltose + Water

FIGURE 4–4

THE FORMATION OF MALTOSE FROM GLUCOSE VIA DEHYDRATION SYNTHESIS

the hot sun or from chemical molecules. Synthesis means putting together, whether it be making a cake from scratch or a larger molecule from smaller subunits. Moreover, dehydration synthesis is not limited to the process by which oligosaccharides are produced from monosaccharides. It is the chemical process by which many large molecules are synthesized or made in an organism.

Speaking of large molecules, there is one additional group of carbohydrates that should be mentioned, namely the *polysaccharides*. Meaning many, *poly* is a prefix used to describe carbohydrates containing many simple sugar units joined together. If you can envision a long string of glucose molecules joined together as in maltose, you are picturing the polysaccharide known as starch. Recall your visits to the carnival or movie theatre. The individual tickets to the rides or shows were dispensed from a single roll containing many tickets joined together. Evidently manufacturing the tickets in a long string proved to be the most efficient way to store them. This same reasoning, therefore, can be applied to why polysaccharides such as starch serve as a convenient way to store energy-rich glucose units. The linking together of sugar units, however, can also provide polysaccharide chains that serve as supporting structures something like the steel rods placed in reinforced concrete. This is the function of such polysaccharides as the cellulose found in plant-cell walls and the component of insects' exoskeletons known as chitin.

LIPIDS To continue with the team introductions for the molecules of life, let's shift our attention to a second member, the lipids. Lipids are a mixed bag of organic chemicals. However, they all share in common the property of being relatively insoluble in water. Recall how difficult it is to remove grease, a lipid, from one's clothing by simply washing with water. Since like dissolves like, water, which is polar, is ineffective in dissolving the nonpolar lipids.

If we can consider the carbohydrates as the team spark plug, then the lipids might very well be considered the team's reserve, or bench, strength. That this is an important role is emphasized by the often quoted comments of a winning coach, "We won because we had superior bench strength." Lipids deserve the name of "super sub" because one of their prime functions is to act as a fuel or energy reserve for the organism. Their efficiency at this role can be seen by comparing the energy yielded by various types of molecules upon burning. Some of these values, measured in units of kilocalories per gram, are recorded in Table 4–2.

TABLE 4–2

Molecule type	Energy yield
carbohydrate	3.74 Kcal/g
lipid	9.3 Kcal/g
protein	3.12 Kcal/g

As you can easily see, weight for weight, lipids yield well over twice as much energy as their companion molecules.

The type of lipids most directly involved with this energy storage function are known as neutral fats. They are formed by chemically combining *fatty acids* with the alcohol *glycerol.* The major structural features of fatty acids are a long chain of carbon atoms bonded to each other and to hydrogens along with an organic acid group known as the *carboxyl,* or –COOH group, as shown in Figure 4–5. Notice the one double bond in oleic acid, which is present in neither palmitic nor stearic acid. Although this difference may seem inconsequential, it is in large measure the explanation for why cooking oils are liquids at room temperature while shortenings are solids. The double bonds make fatty acids *unsaturated,* that is, they do not contain as many hydrogens as they have the potential for. And, as the degree of unsaturation increases in a fat, the tendency to be a liquid at room temperature increases. Such is the case for cooking oil.

In addition to fatty acids, the second component of a neutral fat is glycerol. Glycerol is an alcohol. The alcohol that humans consume from time to time is ethanol, which has the following structure: $CH_3–CH_2–OH$. It is the –OH group, not to be confused with the acidic –COOH group, which determines the compound as an alcohol. The structure of glycerol is

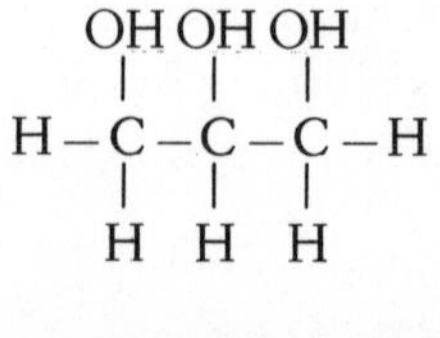

$$\begin{array}{ccccccc} & OH & & OH & & OH & \\ & | & & | & & | & \\ H & - & C & - & C & - & C & - & H \\ & | & & | & & | & \\ & H & & H & & H & \end{array}$$

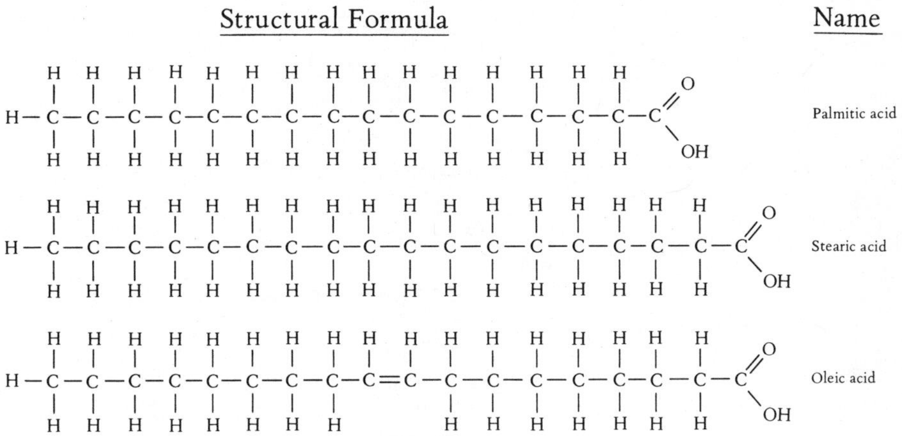

Structural Formula   Name

Palmitic acid

Stearic acid

Oleic acid

FIGURE 4-5

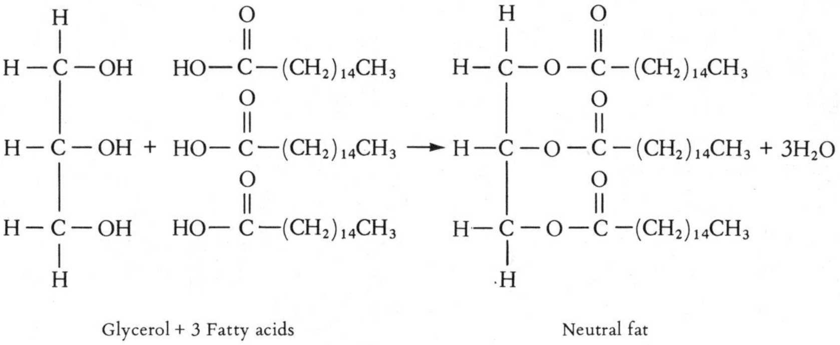

Glycerol + 3 Fatty acids   Neutral fat

FIGURE 4-6

SYNTHESIS OF A FAT

Without question it is an alcohol because it has three OH groups. But don't be tempted to drink it rather than ethanol thinking that it would be three times as powerful. It just doesn't work that way!

From the starting materials of glycerol and fatty acids, then, a fat is synthesized as diagrammed in Figure 4-6. Notice that this reaction involves a dehydration synthesis, that is, one water molecule is removed for each fatty acid tacked on to glycerol.

Because there are no ionic or even polar groups in the fat molecule, it is not surprising that they are not soluble in water. A slightly more complex group of lipids, however, does exhibit some polar properties. These

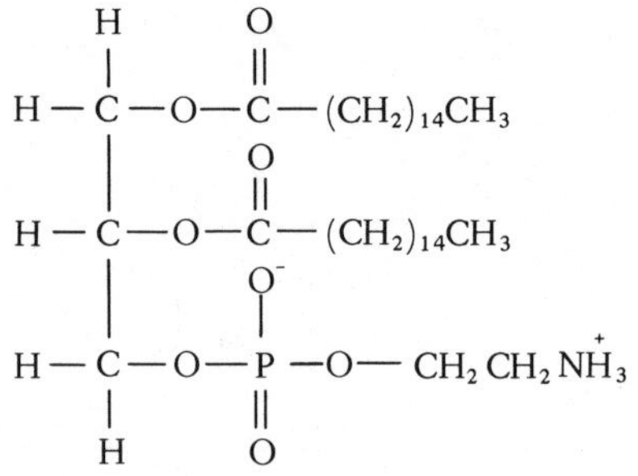

$$
\begin{array}{c}
\text{H}\;\text{O} \\
|\;\;\|\\
\text{H}-\text{C}-\text{O}-\text{C}-(\text{CH}_2)_{14}\text{CH}_3 \\
|\;\text{O} \\
\;\;\|\\
\text{H}-\text{C}-\text{O}-\text{C}-(\text{CH}_2)_{14}\text{CH}_3 \\
|\;\text{O}^- \\
\;\;| \\
\text{H}-\text{C}-\text{O}-\text{P}-\text{O}-\text{CH}_2\,\text{CH}_2\,\overset{+}{\text{N}}\text{H}_3 \\
|\;\|\\
\text{H}\;\text{O}
\end{array}
$$

FIGURE 4–7

PHOSPHATIDYL ETHANOLAMINE

lipids are known as *phospholipids.* One phospholipid, phosphatidyl ethan-olamine, is shown in Figure 4–7. It bears some striking resemblances to a neutral fat, namely it is synthesized from glycerol and it includes two fatty acids. The difference, however, is that the third fatty acid has been replaced by a substituted phosphate group. What is important about this substitu-tion is that it introduces charged groups into the molecule, making one end of it very polar while the rest of the molecule remains nonpolar. This means that one end, the polar end, will be attracted to water while the rest will be repelled. And as we will see in the next chapter, this trait makes phospholipids ideally suited to be structural components of the membranes that act as important boundaries in an organism.

While there are other types of molecules, such as the steroid hormones and certain fat soluble vitamins, that are also classified as lipids, they are beyond the scope of this chapter. Consequently, we will continue with our molecular team introductions by considering next the class of molecules known as proteins.

PROTEINS Proteins, as their name literally indicates, are the topscorers or superstars of our team. The term in Greek means first or number 1. They are of prime importance because they are involved in or control a multitude of different activities. Proteins act as catalysts that control the rates of chemical reactions. It is the presence of protein molecules that allows muscles to contract. The antibodies that the body produces as a means of self-defense are proteins. The chemical "taxi" that carries oxy-gen to wherever it is needed in the body is the protein hemoglobin. Many of the molecules that help regulate the *p*H of the blood are proteins, as are the molecules, like collagen, that provide support for the body. The message, therefore, should be clear. Proteins are indeed the work horses of the team.

As you might suspect from the list above, to be successful in all of these roles, proteins must be rather complex molecules. Like the carbo-

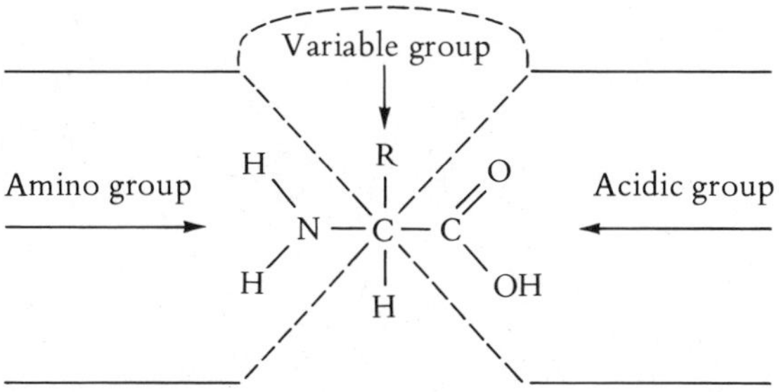

FIGURE 4-8

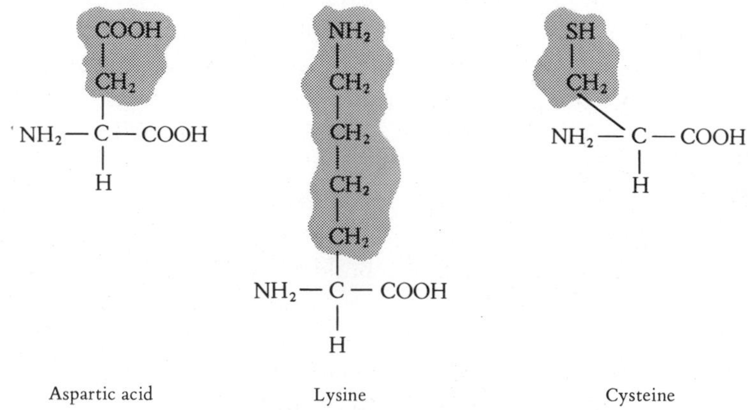

Aspartic acid   Lysine   Cysteine

FIGURE 4-9

hydrates and lipids, proteins contain carbon, hydrogen, and oxygen. In addition, the next most abundant element, nitrogen, is present along with smaller amounts of the element sulfur. These elements are components of organic molecules known as *amino acids,* which serve as the structural building blocks of proteins. The general formula for an amino acid is shown in Figure 4-8. Hopefully, after seeing this formula, the name amino acid loses some of its mystery. *Amino* comes from the $-NH_2$ group, which is known as an amino group; and, as we have seen before, the $-COOH$ or carboxyl group is the functional group of an organic *acid.* Hence the term amino acid. There are approximately 20 different naturally occuring amino acids and all of them have as a common denominator the structures discussed above. The obvious question then becomes, "how do these amino acids differ from one another?" The answer lies with the nature of the group labelled R in the general formula. As indicated, this group is variable, which means that it is different in each different kind of amino acid. Figure 4-9 shows three specific amino acids with their particular R groups shaded.

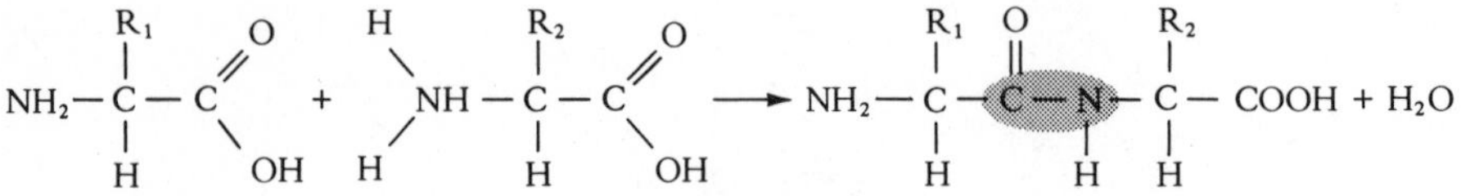

$$NH_2-\overset{\underset{\displaystyle H}{|}}{\underset{}{\overset{\displaystyle R_1}{|}}}\overset{}{C}-\overset{\displaystyle O}{C}\diagdown \quad + \quad \diagup NH-\overset{\underset{\displaystyle H}{|}}{\overset{\displaystyle R_2}{|}}C-\overset{\displaystyle O}{C}\diagdown \quad \longrightarrow \quad NH_2-\overset{\underset{\displaystyle H}{|}}{\overset{\displaystyle R_1}{|}}C-\overset{\displaystyle O}{C}-\overset{\underset{\displaystyle H}{|}}{N}-\overset{\underset{\displaystyle H}{|}}{\overset{\displaystyle R_2}{|}}C-COOH + H_2O$$

FIGURE 4-10

Aspartic acid has an acidic—COOH as part of its *R* side chain. Lysine, on the other hand, has a proton-accepting amino ($-NH_2$) group as part of its side chain, thus making this amino acid basic rather than acidic. Finally cysteine was included to show how the element sulfur can be present in an amino acid, and hence a protein. Rather than worrying about the individual structures, however, the points you should retain are that amino acids differ from one another by virtue of the particular *R* groups that they possess, and that these *R* groups can have quite diverse chemical properties, that is, some can be acidic, others basic, and still others nonpolar.

Having identified the amino acids as the fundamental building blocks of proteins, we must next consider the overall structure of the total building that is the protein itself. Just as a building is constructed in stages or levels, so too total protein structure is composed of various levels of organization. We will mention four levels. The first level, or *primary level,* of organization centers on the way the amino acids are linked together like a string of differently shaped "pop-it" beads. The bonds that join together successive amino acids are known as peptide bonds, one of which is shaded in Figure 4-10. This bond links the carbon atom of the carboxyl group of one amino acid to the nitrogen atom of the amino group of the second amino acid. Two amino acids linked in this way constitute what is known as a *dipeptide.* Proteins, however, contain many amino acids linked together by *peptide bonds,* and thus are known as *polypeptides.* Moreover, just as it is possible to imagine an almost endless number of different strands of "pop-it" beads achieved by altering the numbers and positions of differently shaped beads, so too an almost infinite number of polypeptide chains or proteins can be envisioned by altering the numbers and positions of the twenty different amino acids (see Figure 4-10).

Your picture of a protein molecule at this point is most likely that of a long straight chain of amino acids (Figure 4-11a). While this is an accurate picture to depict the primary level of organization in a protein, the total picture is quite a bit more complicated. Rather than existing as a long straight chain, the linked amino acids are thrown into either coils or pleated sheets. If, as in Figure 4-11b, you picture the "pop-it" beads in our previous discussion as being threaded along a "slinky," you have a coiled arrangement that is one representation of the *secondary level* of organization in

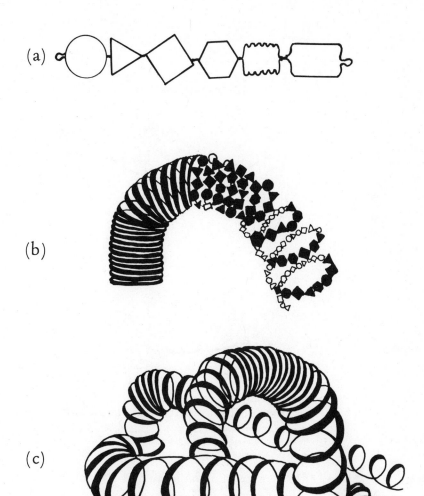

FIGURE 4-11
THE FIRST THREE LEVELS OF PROTEIN STRUCTURE

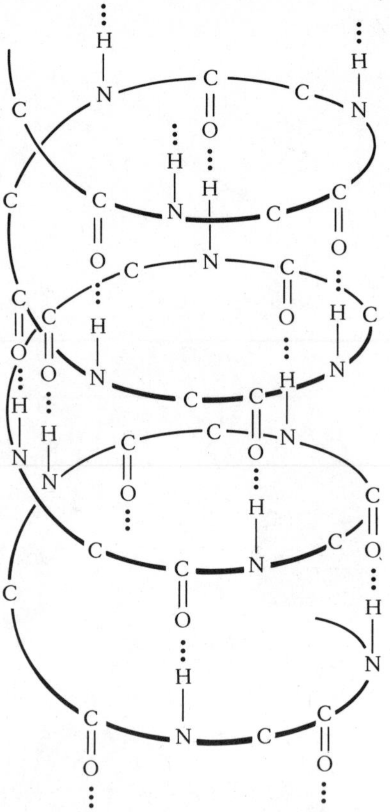

FIGURE 4-12

HYDROGEN BONDS STABILIZING SECONDARY

SECONDARY STRUCTURE J. C. Dearden, *New Scientist* 37, 589.
629, 1968. This first appeared in *New Scientist*, London, the weekly review of
science and technology.

proteins. This coil is known as an *alpha helix* and is stabilized by hydrogen bonding between amino acids in the chain (see Figure 4–12). Moreover, because each individual hydrogen bond is weak it should not be
too surprising that it can easily be disrupted by heat, thereby altering
the three dimensional structure of the protein.

Up to this point we have a chain of amino acids arranged as a coil
or pleated sheet in space. This, however, is still not the complete picture. With our beaded slinky (Figure 4–11c), it is possible to bend or fold
it in places while still retaining some degree of coiling. In a protein this
bending or folding of the chain is known as the *tertiary (third) level* of organization. It is responsible for making the overall protein molecule more
compact, and it causes some of the amino acids present to be buried in the
core of the molecule, while leaving other amino acids exposed on the surface. This tertiary level of organization is maintained by a number of different types of forces including ionic interactions between oppositely
charged acidic and basic amino acids, hydrogen bonding between polar
amino acids, and sulfur bridges between two sulfur-containing amino acids

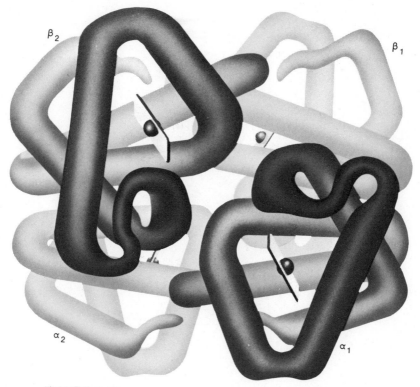

FIGURE 4–13

TERTIARY AND QUARTENARY STRUCTURE OF PROTEINS

Richard E. Dickerson and Irving Geis, *Chemistry, Matter, and the Universe*, copyright © 1978 by The Benjamin/Cummings Publishing Company, Inc. (formerly W. A. Benjamin, Inc.), Menlo Park, California.

known as cysteine. And, since many of these forces are sensitive to changes in hydrogen ion concentration (*p*H), this level of protein structure is also susceptible to change unless the *p*H is maintained constant.

Having described the primary, secondary, and tertiary levels of organization of proteins, we have completed the picture for the simplest of proteins containing a single polypeptide chain. The blood pigment hemoglobin, however, is an example of a protein that contains *four* polypeptide chains. As can be seen in Figure 4–13, the arrangement in space of these four polypeptide chains represents the *fourth or quarternary level* of organization exhibited by proteins. Finally, as we will see in subsequent chapters, it is the complexity and diversity of their structural organization that allows proteins to lay claim to being the superstars of the molecule team of life.

NUCLEIC ACIDS Up to this point then, our team has superstars (protein), reserve strength (lipids), and a spark plug (carbohydrates). Apparently the only ingredient missing is the important role of a captain to

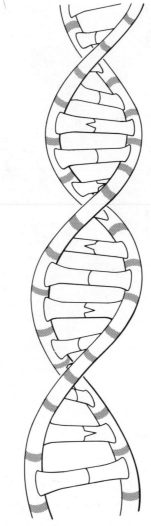

FIGURE 4-14
THE "TWISTED LADDER" OF DNA

direct and control the team's activities. The molecules that fulfill this role on our team are the nucleic acids. One nucleic acid has the play book memorized. This bearer of the cells' genetic information is *deoxyribonucleic acid,* or *DNA* for short. Another nucleic acid that acts as a go-between or messenger for DNA and other cell structures is *ribonucleic acid* or *RNA.* As with many of the other molecules we have discussed in this chapter, especially the proteins, nucleic acids are rather complex molecules composed of many subunits. As Figure 4-14 indicates, DNA is actually double

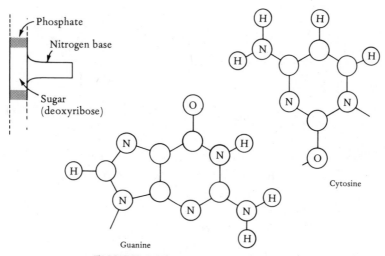

Adenine

Thymine

Phosphate

Nitrogen base

Sugar
(deoxyribose)

Cytosine

Guanine

FIGURE 4-15

COMPONENTS OF A NUCLEOTIDE

stranded, having the overall appearance that can be characterized as a twisted ladder. What are the rungs and side supports of this ladder composed of, that is, what are the basic building blocks of DNA? Unlike the repeating simple sugar units in a polysaccharide or the repetition of a variety of amino acids in a protein, the building blocks of DNA are more complex. Each one, called a *nucleotide,* is composed of a sugar unit, *deoxyribose,* a phosphate group, and finally one of four possible *nitrogenous bases.* The structure of the four bases is shown in Figure 4–15. These bases are *adenine, thymine, cytosine,* and *guanine.* Notice that structur-

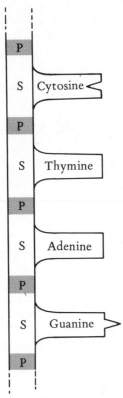

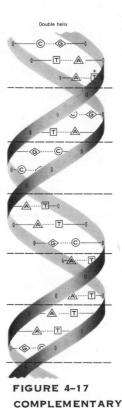

Double helix

FIGURE 4-16

A DNA STRAND SHOWING THE PHOSPHATE AND SUGAR BACKBONE AND THE BASE HALF RUNGS

FIGURE 4-17

COMPLEMENTARY BASE PAIRING IN DNA

Richard E. Dickerson and Irving Geis, *Chemistry, Matter, and the Universe,* Copyright © 1976 by The Benjamin/ Cummings Publishing Company, Inc. (formerly W. A. Benjamin, Inc.), Menlo Park, California.

ally adenine and guanine resemble one another, as do thymine and cytosine. A nucleotide then contains one of these bases joined to a deoxyribose sugar, which is in turn attached to a phosphate group. Successive nucleotides are linked to one another through their sugar and phosphate groups. As Figure 4-16 indicates, therefore, the phosphate-sugar groups form the side supports of one half of the ladder, with the nitrogenous bases of each nucleotide forming a half of each rung. The ladder is completed by adding a second *matching* nucleotide chain as shown on the right in Figure 4-17. Notice the word matching was italicized in the sentence above. The matching is accomplished by the pairs of nitrogenous bases that bond together to form the rungs of the ladder. The bonding is specific rather than haphazard. As can be seen in Figure 4-17, adenine always bonds with thymine and cytosine always bonds with guanine. These four bases are the most important part of the DNA molecule, because the genetic information it contains is coded by the specific sequence of bases that it possesses. As we will see in a later chapter, the bases act as a language that is composed of only four letters A, T, C, and G.

Having discussed DNA, we must next consider RNA. Table 4–3 compares some of the features of DNA and RNA.

TABLE 4-3

Nucleic acid	Number of strands per molecule	Basic building block	Sugar present	Bases present
DNA	2	nucleotides	deoxy-ribose	Adenine Cytosine Guanine Thymine
RNA	1	nucleotides	ribose	Adenine Cytosine Guanine Uracil

As the table indicates both DNA and RNA are composed of nucleotides. RNA, however, is composed of only one rather than two strands. The sugar components mark a second difference between the two acids. The sugar in RNA (*Ribo*nucleic acid) is *ribose* rather than the deoxyribose found in DNA (*Deoxyribo*nucleic acid). Finally, the table points out a third difference. RNA and DNA share three bases in common, adenine, cytosine, and guanine. In RNA, however, *uracil* is the fourth base, replacing thymine.

Since the manner in which the genetic code is transferred from DNA to RNA will be the subject of a later chapter, we can close this one having identified the major players on the molecular team of life. The carbohydrates, lipids, proteins, and nucleic acids are ready. In the next section we will take a look at the condition of the playing field and then be ready for the game itself.

Self-Test

CHAPTER 3   ELEMENTS OF LIFE

1. In addition to oxygen (25 percent), the other two most abundant elements found in living organisms are _____ and _____ .

2. From the following list, identify the properties of carbon that help account for its stability and versatility in living systems.
   a. forms four strong ionic bonds
   b. forms four strong covalent bonds
   c. forms multiple bonds
   d. forms rings and chains with other carbon atoms
   e. bonds only to one other atom

3. An oxygen atom is an avid donor of electrons.
   a. true
   b. false

4a. Which of the following statements is not a characteristic of the water molecule?
   a. The water molecule contains two atoms of hydrogen and one atom of oxygen.
   b. The molecule is polar.
   c. The hydrogen atoms are bent to one side of the molecule and the oxygen is on the other.
   d. All of the atoms in the molecule are arranged in a straight line.

   b. Hydrogen bonds are forces that hold the individual atoms of a water molecule together.
   a. true
   b. false

CHAPTER 4   MOLECULES OF LIFE

1a. Carbohydrate literally means hydrate of carbon because for each carbon atom present in a molecule, hydrogen and oxygen are also present in the same proportions as they are found in water.
   a. true
   b. false

 b. Identify a major role of carbohydrates.
   a. long-term energy storage
   b. bearer of genetic information
   c. catalyst, controlling chemical reactions
   d. immediately available energy source

2. Match the following classes of single sugar molecules with the number of carbon atoms each contains.

Monosaccharide	Number of carbons
pentose	3
triose	4
tetrose	5
hexose	6

3. Because they contain the same number and kinds of atoms but with slightly different structural arrangements, glucose and galactose are said to be isomers of one another.
   a. true
   b. false

4. Maltose contains two glucose units joined together. Maltose, therefore is a(n)
   a. monosaccharide
   b. oligosaccharide
   c. polysaccharide

5. When two molecules are joined together by the addition of a water molecule, this process is called dehydration synthesis.
   a. true
   b. false

6. Starch is a _____ containing many sugar units joined together, and is used primarily as a _____ molecule.

7. The group of organic molecules that are insoluble in polar solvents such as water are known as
   a. carbohydrates
   b. lipids
   c. nucleic acids
   d. proteins

8. The components of a neutral fat are the alcohol, _____, and long-chained _____ acids.

9. Because they are entirely nonpolar, phospholipids are well suited structurally to be components of the cell membrane.
   a. true
   b. false

10a. The class of organic molecules made up from building blocks called amino acids is known as:
   a. carbohydrates
   b. proteins
   c. nucleic acids
   d. lipids

   b. Which of the following is not a function that can be attributed to proteins?
   a. buffer
   b. catalyst
   c. bearer of genetic information
   d. transportation
   e. defense

11. Compare and contrast different amino acids.

12. Match the level of organization found in protein molecules with its appropriate description.

_____ 1. the three dimensional order of separate amino acid chains into one protein molecule

_____ 2. the compact folding and twisting of an amino acid helix in space

_____ 3. a linear sequence of amino acids joined together by peptide bonds

_____ 4. the coiled arrangement of an amino acid chain held together by hydrogen bonds

Level

a. 1st—primary
b. 2nd—secondary
c. 3rd—tertiary
d. 4th—quarternary

13. Identify the principal role of the nucleic acids
a. long-term energy storage
b. bearer of genetic information
c. catalyst, controlling chemical reactions
d. immediately available energy source

14a. A DNA nucleotide is composed of a phosphate group, the sugar *ribose,* and a nitrogen base.
a. true
b. false

b. Draw lines to indicate the specificity in nitrogen base pairing in DNA.
a. adenine
b. guanine
c. cytosine
d. thymine

15. Fill in the following table as a means of comparing and contrasting DNA and RNA.

	Number of strands	sugar	bases present
DNA			
RNA			

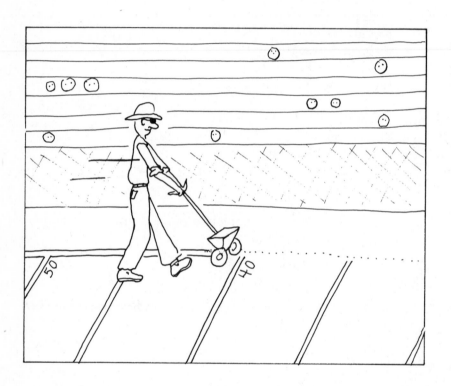

Section Three
THE PLAYING
FIELD

OBJECTIVES FOR SECTION THREE

Chapter 5
LAY OF THE LAND: The Animal Cell

1. Identify five characteristics associated with the living cell.
2. Identify the basic structure and general chemistry of the plasma membrane.
3. Identify the role of diffusion in the functioning of the cell.
4. Distinguish between diffusion and three types of active transport.
5. Identify functions of seven components of the animal cell.

Chapter 6
WARMING UP: Metabolism and Enzymes

1. Distinguish between Catabolism and Anabolism.
2. Identify the role of enzymes in metabolism.
3. Identify the basis for specificity of enzyme activity.
4. Identify the basis of enzyme activity.
5. Identify the activity of seven selected metabolic enzymes.

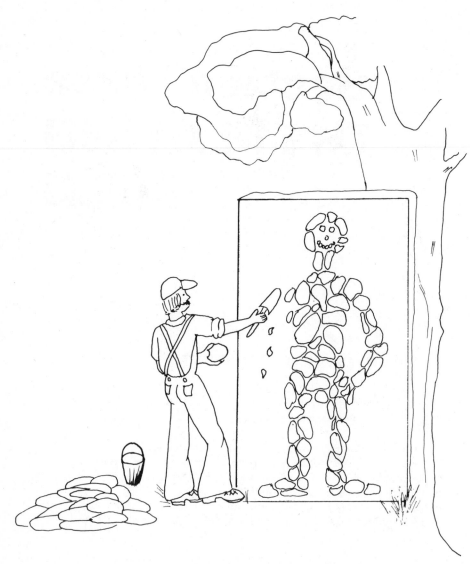

FIGURE 5-1

ASSEMBLING THE PIECES

Chapter 5
LAY OF THE LAND
The Animal Cell

The cartoon character is busily assembling the mosaic figure from pieces that vary in size, shape, and texture. This is symbolic of the variety of materials and structures necessary for life. This is true in terms of the individual cell as well. Along with a description of life and selected activities in the cell, component parts are the major thrust of this chapter.

Actually the word cell was given to the basic unit of life by Robert Hooke in 1665. He was studying the structure of cork and observed many empty areas of similar size. These areas reminded him of monk's rooms in a monastery, which were called cells. However, a living cell is not an empty area. It is alive and exhibits all the characteristics by which we recognize that it is alive. Life is impossible to define; but all living things are relatively easy to recognize and describe.

CHARACTERISTICS OF LIFE Of the many characteristics associated with life we have chosen five for you to learn, and have designed a memory device to help you learn all five with relative ease, shown in Figure 5-2. Now, when you must recall some characteristics of life think of large smelly rats and associate the five initials, each with the appropriate term.

GROWTH refers to the ability of living things to increase in size. Infants grow into larger humans. Seedlings grow into larger plants, and even the wee little bacteria grow. Each of us grows because our cells increase in number and because some cells increase in size. This is true of all multicellular animals and plants, but is not true of the bacteria and most other microorganisms. Unicellular organisms grow only by an increase in cell size.

REPRODUCTION is the ability of living things to increase their numbers. All forms of life we know are offspring produced by existing life forms. Many years ago, 300 or so, it was believed that various animals just

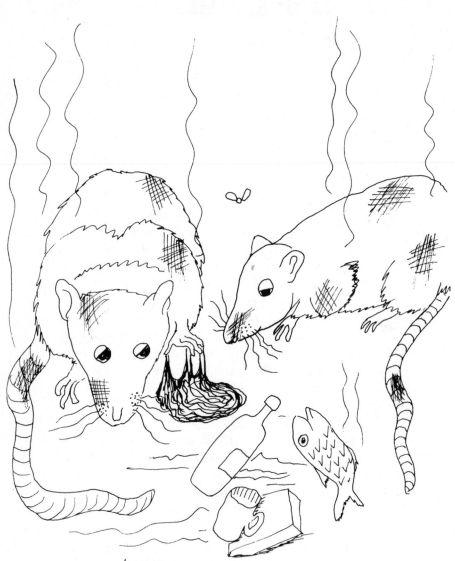

FIGURE 5-2
GIANT RATS HAVE MANY ODORS.

happened. They were created, for example, from decaying food (flies), mud (frogs), or other nonliving materials. It was believed that each was created new and was not the product of a parent or parents.* This kind of mistake is understandable when one realizes that the connection of some parents with their young is often invisible. Ambrose Bierce stated that "Peresilis . . . grew out of the ground where a priest had spilled holy water. Arimaxus was derived from a hole in the earth made by a stroke of lightning. . . . and I have myself seen a man come out of a wine cellar."† This sort of "creation," namely spontaneous generation, that is, life from nonlife, is not reproduction in the sense we choose to use.

HEREDITY refers to the ability of living things to give their offspring their own characteristics: brown eyes, black hair, height, body build. These characteristics are transmitted by way of thousands of bits of information called *genes.* Thus humans produce offspring that are human and not some other animal, and the bacterium called *Streptococcus,* which causes sore throats, produces offspring that are also *Streptococcus.* Some humans also cause a pain in the neck but that doesn't entitle them to be called Streptococcus; they just don't have the right genes.

METABOLISM is the sum total of all chemical reactions necessary for life, that is, the property of life by which cells gain nourishment, build cell structure, and produce energy. The nourishment and energy allow cells to grow, reproduce, and survive. Growth and reproduction require the making of new cell materials for the increases in size and/or numbers. Metabolism furnishes the means to perform these activities.

ORGANIZATION describes the way cells and individuals are put together so that they may function properly. We can take all of the parts of a cell separately; mix them together and we have a mess, not a living cell. A jigsaw puzzle in pieces does not convey the whole picture. The football team in which players do not perform their individual positions according to the game plan will not be successful. Organization implies all of this.

Whatever life is; the five characteristics of life allow us to describe and discuss it. The same characteristics that mean we are alive are also true of plants and microorganisms. Consider the cartoon of the giant smelly rats and think about those properties of life.

CELL PARTS Organization was discussed as a property or characteristic of life in terms of putting all the pieces in the right places. This is true, but organization means a lot more. The pieces have to be there, and each bit must perform activities necessary to life. These activities must be organized and the entire living unit of life must be protected from the environment.

---

*Some microorganisms are capable of reproducing by having one cell split into two, therefore only one parent is required.
†Ambrose Bierce, *The Devil's Dictionary* (New York: Dover Publications, Inc., 1958).

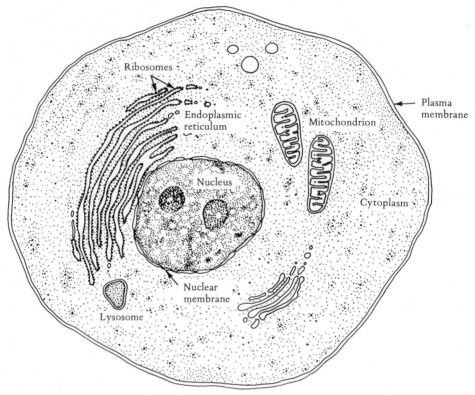

FIGURE 5-3
DIAGRAM OF A TYPICAL ANIMAL CELL

Figure 5–3 shows a typical animal cell. A *plasma membrane* protects each cell in a manner similar to the way the skin protects us. This plasma membrane separates cell stuff from the environment. It allows nourishment to enter and wastes to leave. It has an interesting structure to allow all of this to happen. Picture a pot of soup (see Figure 5–4a). This soup has some pieces of meat, which gradually give off fat that floats on the surface. Eventually the fat forms a thin layer on the surface with pieces of various ingredients floating along with it. Some of the pieces are very small and lie on the surface, while others are bigger and poke through into the soup.

Now picture that pot of soup without the pot in a space vehicle with no gravity (see Figure 5–4b). Without gravity the soup will become a sphere and the fat will completely coat all the fluid. The pieces of floating ingredients will wander all around. This "raft and iceberg" model for the structure of membranes is fairly recent; it states that there are two layers of lipid, and in this lipid "bilayer," protein, lipoprotein, and glycoprotein float like rafts and icebergs. The rafts stay on the surface and the icebergs go down into the water through the surface layers.

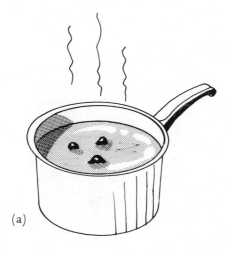

(a)

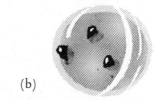

(b)

FIGURE 5-4
MEMBRANE ANALOGY

This membrane is a fairly tough double layer of lipid, and functions as stated before, to protect and allow "things" to go in and out of the cell. How do "things" go into and out of the cell through this supposedly tough membrane? The key to this is the unique chemistry of the lipid bilayer and the protein icebergs. For metabolism, growth, and reproduction to occur, animal cells must be supplied with all of the basic ingredients, including sugars, amino acids, lipids, vitamins, minerals, and oxygen. These can be viewed as wandering around in the fluid outside of the cell. This wandering around is, in essence, *diffusion.* We learn in science that all matter is made up of molecules and that the state of matter—solid, liquid, or gas—depends on how fast the molecules are moving. The slowest movement is in solids and the fastest is in the gases. These movements of water molecules constantly vibrating and hitting the other molecules cause the wandering—the diffusion. Consider a drop of red food coloring in a glass of water. The color spreads until all the water is some shade of pink. Consider a pungent odor escaping from a diaper pail. The odor spreads until the entire room is infiltrated and no corner can escape. The spreading is

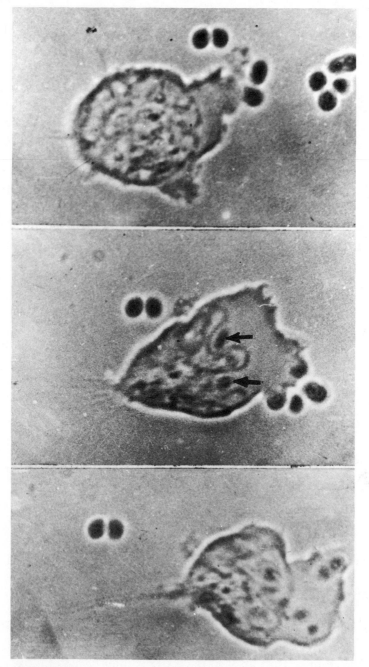

FIGURE 5-5
PHAGOCYTOSIS
W. B. Wood, M. R. Smith, and B. Watson, *Journal of Experimental Medicine*, 84: 387, 1946.

due to diffusion, the movement of a chemical from a high concentration (drop of red color, diaper pail) to a low concentration (clear water, clear air). Thus, diffusion can bring the required nourishment to the membrane of the cell. Diffusion can also account for some of the movement of materials across the membrane into the cell. Some of the materials mix with the lipid bilayer, and others mix with the protein icebergs. Thus these materials diffuse from the higher concentration outside the cell to the lower concentration inside. As the materials inside are used, this keeps the concentration low and more and more will diffuse in. If the concentration equalizes between outside and inside, the diffusion stops. As metabolism occurs, waste products will accumulate and can diffuse out along what is called the concentration gradient: high to less high to low to no concentration of the particular material. One common waste material in animal cells is carbox dioxide (CO_2) produced during the metabolism in which sugars are used to make the energy needed to drive the machinery of the cell.

Unfortunately, all materials needed by the cell cannot simply diffuse through the membrane lipids or protein; some, for example, are too large. In addition, cells often accumulate materials within themselves to concentrations greater than the outside environment. In order to obtain the large molecules or to concentrate materials against the concentration gradient, energy must be expended. This movement of materials requiring energy is called *active transport*. In contrast, the simple diffusion discussed earlier is called *passive transport*.

Animal cells have two processes for bringing large materials in. Amoeba and most of our white blood cells perform *phagocytosis*, literally "cell eating." With phagocytosis amoeba capture food such as other protozoa and bacteria. The white blood cells use phagocytosis to remove invading disease-causing microorganisms from blood and tissue fluids (see Figure 5–5). In addition white blood cells scavenge cell debris—inhaled, ingested, or injected contaminants, whatever they can. The more commonly used process is *pinocytosis*, literally "cell drinking." This involves the taking in of small drops of fluid from the environment with the proteins and other materials dissolved or suspended in them. In an attempt to explain pinocytosis, let's again picture that pot of soup with the layer of fat floating on the surface. Shake the pot and some fat will form droplets in the water. This fat has left the surface, but there is no hole there. Since the lipid layer is fluid it can break and reform quickly and very easily. Sometime when you are cooking a meat soup of some type with fatty meat, for example, chicken with the skin on, spoon off the fat. Notice that the first few times you can remove fat but the layer still covers the surface. Pinocytosis can be pictured as the movement of fluid from outside of the cell to the inside, being trapped in small sacs of lipid membrane (see Figure 5–6). To make these sacs and maintain the integrity of the lipid layer of

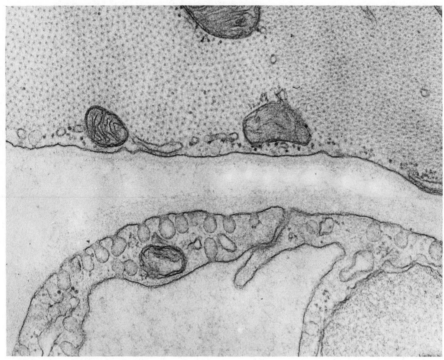

FIGURE 5-6

**PINOCYSTOSIS. ARROWS SHOW MOVEMENT OF
FLUID INTO THE CELL BY MEANS OF FORMATION
OF MEMBRANE SACS.** Fawcett, Don. W., *The Cell, Its Organelles
and Inclusions,* © 1966 by the W. B. Saunders Company, Philadelphia, Pa.

the membrane requires energy. Once inside the cell, the sac disintegrates
and the outside materials are now inside.

Active transport was defined as the movement of materials requiring
energy. Dissolved substances like sugars, amino acids, minerals, and others
that are probably not involved with pinocytosis or phagocytosis need a
means to get into the cell when there is no gradient or that gradient is
higher inside the cell than outside of the cell. This requires a substantial
amount of energy. Compare this with water that flows downhill. No energy is needed to move that water. However, to move that same water uphill
requires energy to run the pump. Water running downhill is equivalent to
passive transport. Pumped water corresponds to active transport.

Nerve cells, for example, require a high concentration of potassium
and a low concentration of sodium for proper functioning. These concentrations are maintained even though outside of the cell is a low concentration of potassium and a high concentration of sodium. It is as if there were
two separate water wheels in the membrane. On one, the buckets will only

hold sodium and on the other, the buckets will only hold potassium. These wheels require energy to collect the sodium or potassium where it is at a low concentration and move it to where it is at a high concentration.

We have been discussing the structure and functioning of the plasma membrane as one of the components of the cell. There are many other components. A total of seven is sufficient for discussion in this chapter on the animal cell* (see Figure 5-3). The seven components are *plasma membrane, cytoplasm, endoplasmic reticulum, ribosome, lysosome, mitochondrion,* and *nucleus.* While discussing the *plasma membrane* we explained that diffusion was occurring outside of the cell. Actually, it is also occurring within fluids of the cell. Materials entering the cell are able to move around inside, so that metabolism will occur. Most of this essential fluid material inside the cell is called *cytoplasm,* literally cell matter. Everything happening within the cell is either in the cytoplasm or in close contact with it.

Endoplasmic reticulum is a complicated way to say a net-like arrangement of membranes in the cytoplasm. These membranes are associated with the synthesis and transport of proteins. These membranes actually separate cytoplasm into compartments in which different activities can take place without interfering one with the other. However, products and reactants can be moved throughout the cytoplasm by these membranes. Materials can, therefore, be moved to wherever needed for the many processes involved in the properties of life.

Membranes of the endoplasmic reticulum are of two types, *smooth* and *rough.* The membranes themselves are smooth. Some, however, have granules attached to make them look roughened. These granules are called *ribosomes,* and they are the particles on which proteins are synthesized from amino acids. More information about ribosomes and protein synthesis is given in Chapter 8.

Earlier we described activities of the cell membrane—phagocytosis and/or pinocytosis—that can bring into the cell materials too large for passive transport through the membrane. Once these materials, such as some proteins, fats, and carbohydrates, enter the cell, they must be processed. In the same manner, hunks of meat, potatoes, and candy bars must be processed in our digestive system so that the essential nutrients can be used for our metabolism, growth, and reproduction. In the individual cell, this processing is accomplished by a cell structure called a *lysosome,* literally, a digesting body.

---

*The animal cell is identified in biology as a **eucaryote.** This means, in essence, that there are membranes in the cytoplasm. In contrast, the procaryote type of cell has few if any internal membranes. Bacteria and blue green algae are the only examples of procaryotes. All other forms of life are eucaryotes. Viruses, having no true membranes of their own, are often classified as nonliving.

Lysosomes are membranous sacs that contain unique proteins capable of performing activities such as producing amino acids from proteins and simple sugars from polysaccharides. These special proteins that are able to perform the digestive processes are called *enzymes*. We will say more about enzymes in the next chapter; however, it is important to mention that enzymes are capable of many more kinds of activities than taking large molecules apart. Lysosomes sort of "float" in the cytoplasm and are able to join with membrane sacs containing materials brought in by phagocytosis and/or pinocytosis. Thus joined, the lysosomes' enzymes digest the materials that were brought in. Subsequently, the membranes of the lysosomes disintegrate and all the digested materials are literally in the soup.

One other kind of membrane structure found floating in the cytoplasm is the *mitochondrion* (plural:mitochondria), which literally means thread. Mitochondria are really special structures containing enzymes necessary for converting sugars into energy. They can be thought of as electric power plants, for as long as appropriate fuels are brought to them, energy is generated. We can store electricity in batteries; mitochondria store energy in a special chemical called *ATP*. More about energy and ATP in Chapter 7.

The last cell component of concern here is the *nucleus*. The word means kernel or seed, literally the central part or core of something. Often nucleus is used, as in the case of an organization, to imply those individuals who are most important to that organization. In the cell, the nucleus is the component that serves as the control center for all or nearly all of the large number of activities associated with life. The information needed by the cell to make all of the structures and perform all of the activities is contained in a chemical composing the units of heredity we previously referred to as genes. The DNA is found in the *nucleoplasm* or nuclear matter, which is surrounded by a double membrane known as the *nuclear membrane*. These membranes have openings or pores allowing the necessary movement of materials into and out of the nucleus. These activities will be described in more detail in Chapter 8.

The basic structures of the living cell are important to an understanding of life and its many varied characteristics. One of these characteristics, metabolism, is discussed in more detail in the remaining chapters of this book.

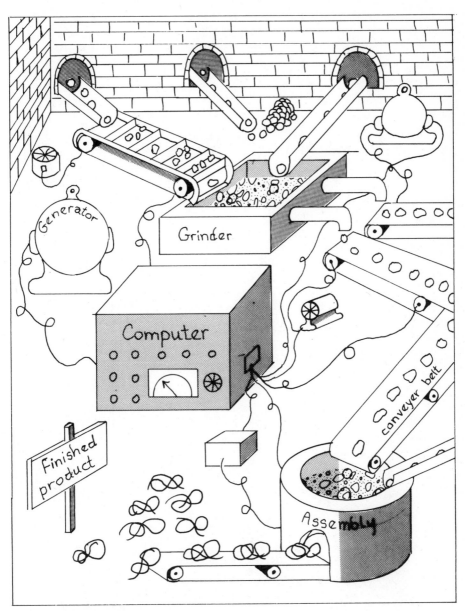

FIGURE 5–7

THE CELL AS A FACTORY. CAN YOU FIND THE FOLLOWING CELL COMPONENTS IN THIS FACTORY: PLASMA MEMBRANE, CYTOPLASM, ENDOPLASMIC RETICULUM, RIBOSOME, LYSOSOME, MITOCHONDRIM, NUCLEUS?

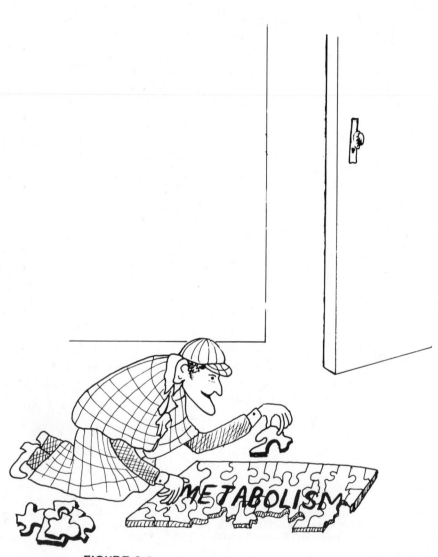

FIGURE 6-1

"ELEMENTARY, MY DEAR . . ."

Chapter 6
WARMING UP
Metabolism and Enzymes

Slowly, but surely, we are presenting all the various pieces of the puzzle called metabolism. In this chapter we will build on the framework of the previous chapters in an attempt to tie together various rules, players, and conditions for playing the game. In addition we are concentrating on some basics of metabolism and in particular the most unique materials: *enzymes.*

METABOLISM

Metabolism has been defined, simply, as the chemical activities of life: all of the various processes by which you obtain energy, grow, heal, think, feel, and dispose of waste materials.

CATABOLISM AND ANABOLISM Metabolism is divided into two broad categories: *catabolism* and *anabolism.* Catabolism is often called the portion of metabolism involved with the breaking down of complex organic molecules into simpler molecules. During this process of taking molecules apart, energy is released, and that includes the heat to keep us warm.

The energy and simpler molecules produced in catabolism can thus be used in anabolism. Anabolic reactions deal with the building up or synthesis of complex molecules from specific building blocks. Thus catabolism produces energy and building materials to be used in anabolism to make cell components and allow the cell to do work.

To illustrate this, let's picture a big baked potato. A good deal of the potato is starch, as you know, a polysaccharide. During catabolic reactions the starch is broken into the disaccharide, maltose, and finally into glucose units. Some of the glucose units continue in catabolism through additional reactions, which produce carbon dioxide, water, and energy. Now there are glucose units and energy available for anabolism. Some energy will be used to combine glucose units into polysaccharides characteristic of our cells. The potato plant used a set of enzymes to combine glucose units into starch during anabolism. We use different enzymes with glucose and make a polysaccharide called glycogen, among others.

In our brief discussion of catabolism and anabolism only starch was mentioned as a source of cell materials and energy. All metabolism requires many different types of raw materials to perform all the varied activities of life. In Chapters 3 and 4 you learned of this chemistry of life, in general, and the major large organic molecules, in particular. Proteins, carbohydrates, lipids, and nucleic acids make up the structural and functional components of the cell, and also serve as the sources of our own components. Energy is required for the synthesis of these materials from basic building blocks. Why go to all the trouble of eating good beef protein, digesting it, and then have to put the amino acids back together to make protein? It seems wasteful of time and energy. Wasteful or not, we cannot absorb beef protein and use it to make our cell membranes. Also, remember that most people consume beef protein cooked, and cooking denatures protein so that it is not functional. In any case, we must break down—catabolize—dietary protein to component amino acids, and subsequently synthesize—anabolize—the amino acids to make our own proteins. Cell membranes, chromosomes, ribosomes all require protein; uniquely ours. In addition, enzymes are primarily proteins, and by the end of this chapter you will know why enzymes are so very significant in cell metabolism.

MINERALS AND VITAMINS Minerals and vitamins are required by cells in very small quantities often called trace amounts. Minerals were described previously as being inorganic and having particular functions essential to life. For example, iron is necessary for blood to be able to carry oxygen, and calcium is required for bones, teeth, and cell membrane activities. Vitamins, on the other hand, are organic, and as a rule function with the protein portion of some enzymes to allow the enzyme to do whatever the enzyme is supposed to do. More about this very soon.

A very simple experiment performed in 1881 showed that something in the diet other than purified carbohydrate, protein, fat, and minerals is necessary to sustain life. Animals were fed this artificial diet and did not thrive. Thus something vital to life was required. The name vitamin can be interpreted to mean "life giving chemical."

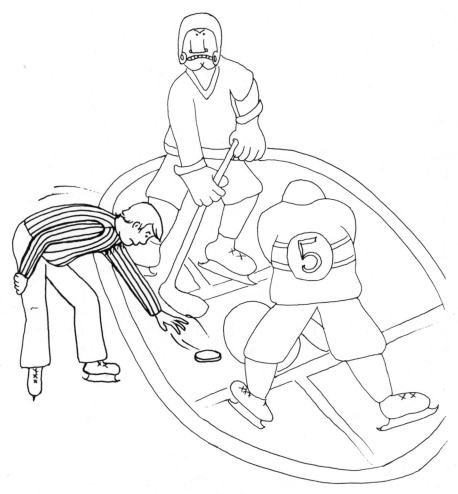

FIGURE 6-2
THE REFEREE TRIGGERS THE ACTION.

ENZYMES The word enzyme has popped up a number of times so far in this book. What actually is an enzyme? What does it do? Why is it considered so very important? Enzymes allow the chemical reactions of metabolism to occur. In the cartoon shown in Figure 6–2, you see two burly hockey players waiting to go to work. They cannot play the game until the referee puts the puck into action. The referee represents the enzyme that allows the players or chemicals to react. One key word describing enzymes is *compatible.* Enzymes function, do their thing, under conditions compatible with life. Your body temperature varies over a few degrees in different areas but is generally accepted to be 98.6° Fahrenheit which is 37° Celsius or Centigrade. Your *p*H or acid concentration varies considerably in parts of the body—about 1–2 in the stomach and 7–8 in the small intestine; however, most tissue fluids are at 7.4 You may wish to review the discussion on pH in Chapter 2. Enzymes in these various tissues function best at a particular temperature and pH level. Slight changes from the normal will only slightly change the activity of the enzymes. Significant changes in temperature or pH can alter the shape of the enzyme and destroy its activity. Next time you boil or poach an egg, watch what happens to the egg white as it is heated. The color changes and the consistency becomes thicker and more solid. The heating has changed the shape of the protein by forcing a reaction between portions of the protein and the water. The effect of acid on protein can also be tested easily in the kitchen. Take a small amount of milk, add some vinegar, and stir. If nothing happens in a few moments add a little more vinegar and continue stirring. Sometime soon the milk will form clumps of milk protein called curds, and you have just made cottage cheese. The acid caused shape changes in the milk protein.

Enzymes are often defined as *organic catalysts;* substances that enable reactions to occur under milder conditions than in the absence of the substance. The particular substance, although taking part in the reaction, is not changed, permanently, by the reaction and allows the reaction to occur at a faster, more *controlled* rate. Thus we have special substances, enzymes, which allow chemical reactions to proceed at a faster, controlled rate under conditions compatible with life. The word itself comes from the Greek *enzymos* for leavening, or a substance that can cause dough to rise. In making breads and pastries, the ingredients are mixed and the dough is allowed to rise. What happens is that carbon dioxide is being made in the dough, and the gas makes the dough expand just as a balloon expands as you blow into it. Yeast is a common source of leavening, since these microorganisms, by means of enzymes, are able to make carbon dioxide from sugar in the dough. Next time you take a slice of bread, examine the texture and look for the little holes which are the sliced bubbles made by the gas during leavening.

The conversion of sugar into gas by yeast is an interesting kitchen experiment. Take a glass with a few ounces of sugar water and add a small amount of bakers yeast. The sugar water can be made by dissolving a teaspoon of sugar in 2–3 ounces of warm water (not hot). After adding the yeast let the glass sit for a few hours and usually within that time gas bubbles will begin to rise from the yeast which have settled to the bottom. Just as bakers do not always use yeast for leavening, you can perform the experiment with baking soda and vinegar. Take a few ounces of vinegar in a glass and sprinkle in a little baking soda. Almost immediately carbon dioxide gas bubbles will form. The acid condition, caused by acetic acid in vinegar, decreases the amount of carbon dioxide that can dissolve in the water and the extra gas comes out as bubbles. Small toy rockets have been designed to use baking soda and vinegar for propulsion. In the right condition these two ingredients produce quite a thrust by the sudden formation of the carbon dioxide.

Although the yeast and the toy rocket both produce carbon dioxide, this is where the similarity ends. The yeast use enzymes to produce carbon dioxide because they, like most other life forms, cannot metabolize under conditions that are as acidic as vinegar.

Consider also the energy output of both exercises. Baking soda and vinegar produce sufficient energy to power the rocket. Yeast and sugar produce sufficient energy to make new yeast cells and some heat. In the rocket, rapid energy production is required. In the yeast cells, rapid energy production would be lethal. Living cells require steady availability of energy, much in the same way that a battery supplies electricity on demand. Recall that the animal cell has mitochondria to make ATP or stored energy. Yeast need the same thing.

Another characteristic of enzymes is their *specificity*, that is, their ability to perform one particular reaction or kind of reaction. A chemical analysis is called specific if it yields a particular reaction with one particular substance. There are several tests for diabetes in which urine is checked for the amount of sugar present. The sugar of concern is glucose. One test in which a tablet is placed in a test tube with urine produces a color change if glucose or a similar sugar is present. Another test involves wetting a paper strip with urine. A color change here tells you that there is glucose in the urine. Both tests are specific, but the second one is the more specific: the latter reaction occurs only when glucose is in the urine. The reason for the high degree of specificity is the use of an enzyme which will produce only the given reaction with glucose. *Faster, controlled, compatible,* and *specific* are a set of key words describing enzymes.

Metabolic reactions occur in a step-wise fashion. Often each step occurs because of a different enzyme. If enzymes were not specific the activities of cells would be much more difficult to control. What exactly accounts for this specificity? Probably the best analogy is the lock and key. One key will open one particular lock because the key has grooves, bumps, and edges which depress certain structures in the lock to cause it to open. One groove in the wrong place and the key doesn't work. In our analogy the key corresponds to the enzyme and the lock is symbolic of the substance to be changed: the *substrate.* Substrate means the materials of which something is made. Thus in the diabetes test for glucose, the glucose is the substrate and the changed glucose results in the color reaction. In the earlier exercise with yeast and sugar, the sugar was the first substrate.

Now, back to specificity. It may be difficult to imagine protein as having the kind of rigid structure we think of as a key. Well, yes and no.

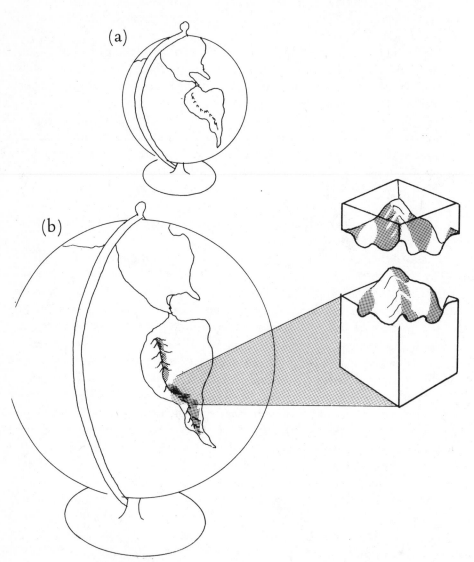

FIGURE 6-3
GLOBAL ANALOGY FOR ENZYME SPECIFICITY

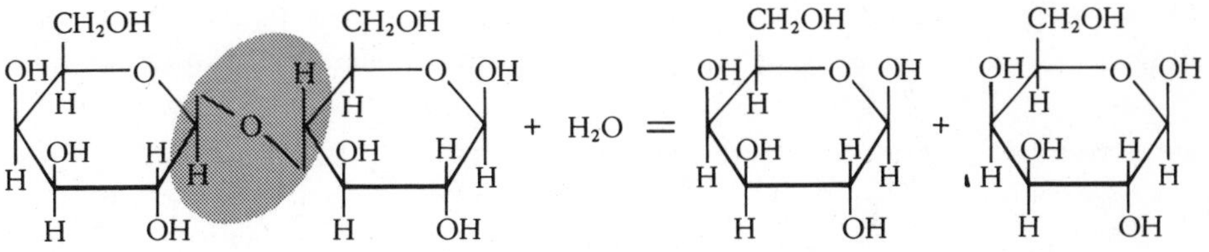

Lactose   +   Water   =   Glucose   +   Galactose

FIGURE 6–4

In Chapter 4 you learned that protein can have as many as four levels of organization. Enzymes are composed of proteins which are folded and bent into a rather compacted form and generally called globular protein. The word *globe* implies a good deal more than the fact that these proteins are sort of rounded. Our planet is a globe (see Figure 6–3a). Consider a plastic model of the earth, which includes an accurate representation of the mountains, valleys, canyons, deserts, and the depths of the oceans, without the water. From a distance the model is sort of round with various colors and shadings. As you get closer, more and more details are evident. Some mountains are taller and rougher, some valleys are narrower, shaped differently, and so forth. Even closer you find caves in the mountains and some irregularities in the terrain. This is similar to what an enzyme looks like. Now picture a particular part of the model (see Figure 6–3b) and pour some plaster of Paris over it. When the plaster is set and removed, examine the casting you have just made, theoretically. Where the hills are found on the globe, a valley is located in the cast. The casting fits onto and into the globe just as a substrate fits onto and into the correct enzyme. That is specificity.

You know that enzymes allow chemical reactions to occur faster and in a controlled manner and to be compatible with conditions necessary for life while being highly specific. You also know why enzymes are specific. If a substrate cannot fit with the enzyme there can be no activity to allow a reaction to occur.

Let's look at our enzyme-substrate model and discuss what is meant by enzyme activity. We have a globe and a piece of plaster that fits onto a portion of that globe (see Figure 6–3b). Every enzyme has an area that is called the *active site*. The particular activity of the enzyme occurs here. Let's picture the plaster as a molecule of milk sugar or lactose and the globe will be the enzyme (lactase) that can cause lactose to become one molecule of glucose and one of galactose, another monosaccharide (Figure 6–4). Examine the circled portion of the lactose molecule. In order to separate the two monosaccharides, all that is necessary is to add one molecule of water (H$_2$O or HOH) across this bond. This is the part of the lactose molecule which is in contact with the active site of the enzyme and causes one side to pick up H and the other side to get OH, yielding glucose and galactose, the products of the reaction.

Our model lactose is labeled to show you which part is glucose and which is galactose; note that the bond that must be broken will rest in the active site of the enzyme. When the lactose settles into the right position, various atoms exert pushes and pulls on the lactose to create some stress at the bond to be broken. The bond will open and H and OH will react immediately. When this happens the molecules do not fit as well and they leave the enzyme. The active sites of some enzymes are part of the protein; however, other enzymes have two or even three components. The protein portion of the complex enzyme is called an *apoenzyme* and must be joined by a smaller organic molecule, the *coenzyme.* Chemical analysis of coenzymes has shown that the vitamins we discussed briefly earlier in the chapter are involved in their structure. Some enzymes also require minerals or trace elements. For example, several enzymes you use to get energy from glucose require magnesium, and the enzyme that starts to break down starch in your saliva requires chloride.

Another factor that affects enzyme activity is the concentration of substrate and product. Remember, a substrate plus the enzyme for that substrate under appropriate conditions will result in one or more products. Lactose + lactase yields glucose + galactose. In this example the lactase can also make lactose from glucose and galactose. The enzyme is called *reversible.* In that case glucose and galactose become substrates and lactose is the product. Instead of breaking a bond and putting a molecule of water in, now the same enzyme can remove a molecule of water and produce lactose. The enzyme "knows" which activity to perform—forward or backward—depending on whether there is more lactose to be split or more glucose and galactose to be combined.

NAMING ENZYMES A generally accepted method for naming enzymes is to take the name of the substrate and add the suffix *-ase* to all or part of the name. Lactase is the enzyme that splits lactose. Since lactose is a carbohydrate, lactase is broadly classified as a carbohydrase. Thus an enzyme that affects protein is a protease and an enzyme that affects lipids, that is, fats and oils, is called lipase. These three categories: *carbohydrase, protease,* and *lipase* are used for enzymes that usually function in catabolic reactions. When the cell synthesizes its own DNA which is a *polymer,* for example, the enzyme *polymerase* puts the basic units or nucleotides together to form the DNA. We want you to know three more kinds of enzymes to help you understand the materials of the next two chapters. They are *dehydrogenase, deaminase,* and *decarboxylase.*

The prefix *de-* means "from" and implies that something is removed from the substrate. The mid-portion of the name tells you what is being removed. Hydrogen, an amino group, and a carboxyl group are the chemicals of particular concern. Hydrogen you have heard about frequently in these chapters. Amino and carboxyl groups were discussed in Chapter 4 as being primary components of amino acids. Carboxyl groups are also important in fatty acids. Thus a deaminase is an enzyme that removes an amino group. The amino group, $-NH_2$ is given another H by the enzyme and becomes ammonia, NH_3. A decarboxylase is an enzyme that removes a carboxyl group. The carboxyl group, $-COOH$ loses an H because of the enzyme and becomes carbon dioxide, CO_2.

This chapter has dealt with enzymes and their role in catabolism and anabolism. The last section of this book explores these activities in more detail. Chapter 7 deals with catabolism, while Chapter 8 deals with anabolism and how enzymes can be controlled within the cell.

Self-Test

CHAPTER 5 LAY OF THE LAND

1. List and describe, briefly, the five characteristics of life presented in Chapter 5.

2. The plasma membrane is primarily a _____ bilayer in the middle with _____ on both surfaces. In addition some _____ stick all the way through.

3. How does diffusion assist in the functioning of a cell?

4. Diffusion is a type of _____ transport.
   a. active
   b. passive

5. Active transport differs from passive transport chiefly in the fact that active transport requires _____ to move materials across the plasma membrane while passive transport does not.

6. Pinocytosis is considered a type of active transport.
   a. true
   b. false

7. List and describe, briefly, three types of active transport.

8. Match the functions on the left with the cell components on the right.

    ____1. contains all information for cell to function   a. plasma membrane
    ____2. particles on which proteins are synthesized   b. lysosome
    ____3. protect cell from the environment and serve   c. cytoplasm
    _____ to allow food in and wastes out   d. nucleus
    ____4. separates cytoplasm into compartments and   e. mitochondrion
    _____ transports materials through the cell   f. ribosome
    ____5. digests materials brought in from outside   g. endoplasmic
    ____6. produces energy for cell   reticulum
    ____7. primarily fluid material in cell in which chemical activities take place

CHAPTER 6 WARMING UP

1. What is the difference between catabolism and metabolism?

2. In metabolism, enzymes:
   a. cause different reactions to occur
   b. change the body's pH
   c. speed up the body's existing reactions but greatly increase body temperature in doing so.
   d. speed up the body's existing reactions without greatly increasing body temperature
   e. more than one of the above is true

3. What accounts for enzyme specificity?

4. What portion of an enzyme is responsible for enzyme activity?
   a. globular portion
   b. substrate
   c. compatible portion
   d. active site
   e. reactive portion

5. What are the functions of the following types of enzymes?
   a. carbohydrase
   b. protease
   c. lipase
   d. polymerase
   e. dehydrogenase
   f. deaminase
   g. decarboxylase

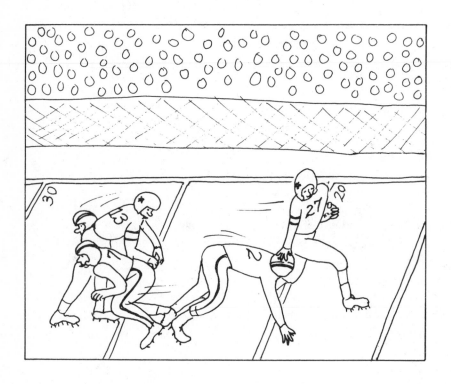

Section Four
THE GAME

OBJECTIVES FOR SECTION FOUR

Chapter 7
BREAKDOWN: Catabolism and Energy

1. Define energy and list examples of its use in the cell.
2. Discuss the appropriateness of ATP as the cell's energy currency.
3. Describe two modes of ATP production.
4. Identify for carbohydrates, the three major sequences of reactions involved with ATP production and the location of each in the cell.
5. Identify for glycolysis (a) major chemical reactants; (b) activity of triosephosphate isomerase; (c) use and production of ATP; (d) points of reduced NAD production.
6. Identify the uses of reduced NAD in anaerobic systems.
7. Identify, for the transition reaction and Krebs citric acid cycle, the following information relating to products from a single glucose molecule: (a) major chemical reactants; (b) numbers of carbons lost as carbon dioxide; (c) numbers of reduced coenzymes, NAD and FAD; (d) numbers of ATP produced by substrate phosphorylation.
8. Identify for the electron transport system: (a) major electron acceptors in sequence; (b) points of ATP production; (c) numbers of ATP produced per electron pair from either NAD or FAD as the initial step in the system.
9. Use your knowledge of the numbers of ATP produced by each of the three major sequences of reactions described above, to contrast the efficiency of energy production in an aerobic vs. an anaerobic system.
10. Link protein and fat subunits to energy production in the three energy sequences described above.

Chapter 8
BUILD UP: Protein Synthesis and Control of Enzyme Activity

1. Describe the "one gene, one protein" theory and use it to explain a mechanism by which an information molecule such as DNA could control the structure and function of an entire cell.
2. Describe the language of the genetic code in terms of the following: triplet, nonoverlapping, degenerate, redundant.
3. Demonstrate your knowledge of the method of m-RNA production known as transcription.
4. Demonstrate your knowledge of the mechanism of protein synthesis by describing the processes of translation.
5. Describe two levels at which the cell is able to control enzyme activity.
6. Describe the operon model of the transcription level of control of enzyme activity.
7. Describe the feedback inhibition model of the substrate level of control of enzyme activity.

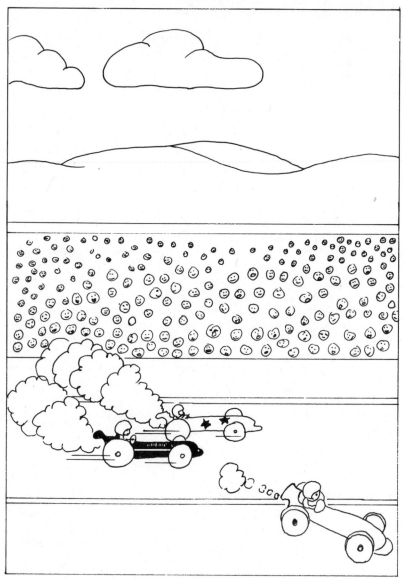

FIGURE 7-1

RUNNING OUT OF GAS

Chapter 7
BREAKDOWN
Catabolism and Energy

ENERGY

The white car is leading the race seconds away from the checkered flag and victory (Figure 7-1). Suddenly the car glides to a stop only to be left in the exhaust fumes of the ultimate victor. What is the explanation for this not uncommon sight in racing circles? A tremendous amount of work must be done to move a race car at breathtaking speeds around and around a race track. Since the ability to do work to move a force through a distance is defined as *energy,* a successful race car must necessarily expend large amounts of energy. The source of energy for the race car, of course, is the fuel it burns. Evidently our white car must have expended its entire energy supply, converting it into motion and heat. It stopped because it ran out of its energy supply, the fuel, and consequently could no longer do any work.

USAGE IN ORGANISMS How does this analogy apply to living organisms? To continue to run, that is, live, we must do work. Fibers in our muscle cells move resulting in muscular contraction. Cells in our endocrine glands synthesize and export hormones, electrical impulses speed along our nerve fibers, kidneys efficiently filter our blood. All of these processes are forms of work, which require an expenditure of energy. What then is our energy source and how do we avoid the "empty tank syndrome" of our race car? Our energy comes from the food that we eat. The carbohydrates, fats, and proteins we consume have a vast wealth of energy locked into the chemical bonds of which they are constructed. Therefore, a continued intake of appropriate amounts of foodstuffs assures us of constant supply of energy.

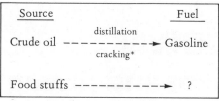

*Cracking: splitting large hydrocarbons into smaller ones in order to reduce boiling point.

FIGURE 7–2
CONVERSION TO FUEL

CONVERSION TO USABLE FORM The situation, however, is not quite as simple as our last statement might have you believe. The foodstuffs that we eat, for example, are not quite analogous to the gasoline used as fuel for a car's engine. Rather they are more like crude oil that is taken from the ground. To see why, let us consider Figure 7–2.

Crude oil, although containing much energy, is not in a form that can be efficiently used by a car's engine, thus the need for the refining process shown in Figure 7–2. In the living organism, foodstuffs are analogous to the crude oil. They, like the oil, contain much energy, but in a form not readily usable by the cells of the organism. What then is necessary to complete Figure 7–2? How are the energy-rich foodstuffs "refined" in the cell and what is the usable energy source produced by this process? These are the questions we will address in the remainder of this chapter.

ATP STRUCTURE The cell's energy source, which is analogous to gasoline, is a molecule known as adenosine triphosphate and referred to most frequently as *ATP*. Figure 7–3 shows the chemical structure of this molecule.

Some of the subunits of this molecule should be familiar to you from our earlier discussion of important organic molecules. You should recall adenine as one of the nitrogenous bases found in all nucleic acids; and ribose as the sugar component of Ribonucleic acids (RNA). An adenine-ribose complex is called adenosine. The remainder of the molecule is the triphosphate portion, named for the three phosphate groups that it contains. Notice the two bonds represented by the squiggly lines between the phosphate groups. It is these bonds which, as we will see shortly, make ATP such an attractive candidate for the fuel molecule to be used by the cells as its immediate energy currency.

PROPERTIES OF ATP What properties should such a molecule possess? First of all, it must be able to be utilized as quickly and easily by the cell as gasoline is by a car's engine. Moreover, when consumed, it should yield

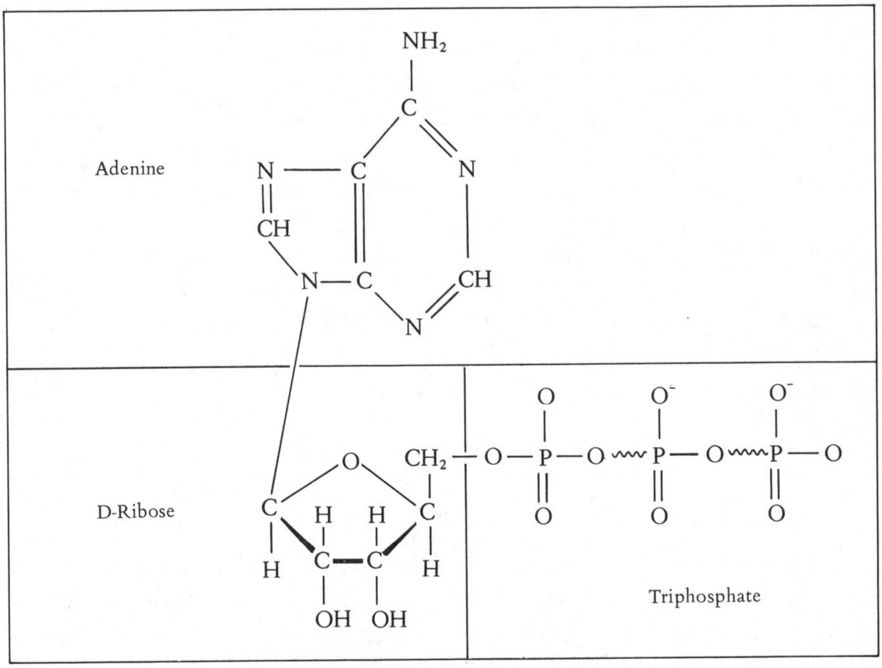

FIGURE 7-3
STRUCTURE OF ATP

the right amount of energy, that is it shouldn't contain so much energy that a great deal will be wasted, or so little that it is inadequate to drive a reaction. Also, the energy source should be one that can take part in a wide variety of reactions all over the organism. It shouldn't be so specialized, in either structure or location, that its use would be limited. Finally, our energy source should be something that the cell produces in abundance and can regenerate just about as quickly as it is consumed.

ATP USAGE Let's see now how ATP exhibits some of these properties. If you refer back to Figure 7–3, you'll see that four of the oxygen atoms of the phosphate groups have negative charges. This is because oxygen gains an electron when it is disassociated from hydrogen, with which it is usually found. However, since like charges repel one another and since in ATP there are four negative charges relatively close to one another, extra energy is required to overcome this repulsion and hold the molecule together. Thus, when the terminal phosphate bond, represented by the squiggly line in Figure 7–3, is broken by an enzyme, a large amount of energy is made available to do the cell's work. It is for this reason that the terminal bond in ATP is termed a *high energy bond*. This reaction is symbolized in Figure 7–4.

In this reaction *adenosine triphosphate (ATP)* is converted to *adenosine diphosphate (ADP)* and *inorganic phosphate (Pi)*. Moreover, as the figure indicates, a sizable amount of energy, approximately 7–8 kilocalories, is released quickly and easily. But best of all, this amount of energy is approximately the amount needed to drive a variety of energy requiring processes with a minimum of energy being dissipated as heat.

ATP REGENERATION One criterion mentioned for the molecule that is to act as the cell's energy currency is that it can be regenerated quickly and easily after it is consumed. Here again ATP fits the bill, because it can be regenerated via a number of different chemical reactions. All of these reactions, however, fall into one of two general categories as outlined in Figure 7–5.

In Figure 7–5, reaction (a) is an example of a mode of synthesis termed *substrate level phosphorylation*. In this type of reaction an energy-rich food intermediate is further decomposed releasing energy that can be used to bind a phosphate on to ADP, thereby producing energy-rich ATP. Reaction (b) is actually a summary of a series of specific reactions termed the electron transport system, during which the energy yielded by the oxidation of a coenzyme such as $NADH_2$ is employed to link an inorganic phosphate group (P_1) to ADP. Since the energy used to drive this reaction is derived from the oxidation of a coenzyme, this mode of ATP production is termed *oxidative phosphorylation*.

CARBOHYDRATE CATABOLISM

Remember, however, that not only is it advantageous for ATP to be produced in a variety of ways, but it must also be produced in abundance. In one particular sequence of processes in the cell a single molecule of the carbohydrate glucose can be "refined" to produce thirty-eight* molecules of ATP. Since this sequence accounts for a very large percentage of the total ATP produced, we will devote much of the remainder of this chapter to this particular topic.

Figure 7–6 identifies the major sequences of reactions by which carbohydrates are "refined" to produce ATP and their intracellular locations. Glucose is initially degraded or refined by a series of reactions known as *glycolysis*, with the enzymes responsible for this sequence of reactions being located in the cell cytoplasm (Figure 7–6a). The actual yield of ATP during the glycolytic process is minimal. However, another end product of glycolysis is *pyruvic acid*. This compound can be modified by what is called the *transition reaction* so that it can enter the fluid matrix of the mitochondrion and thereby be available for the next sequence of reactions

---

*Later in this chapter you will learn that all cells do not produce thirty-eight ATP's.

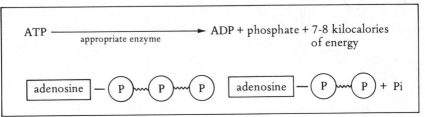

ATP $\xrightarrow[\text{appropriate enzyme}]{}$ ADP + phosphate + 7-8 kilocalories of energy

adenosine — (P) ⌇ (P) ⌇ (P)   adenosine — (P) ⌇ (P) + Pi

FIGURE 7-4

ENERGY RELEASE FROM ATP

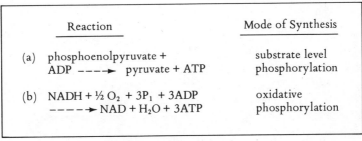

Reaction	Mode of Synthesis
(a) phosphoenolpyruvate + ADP $\dashrightarrow$ pyruvate + ATP	substrate level phosphorylation
(b) NADH + ½ O$_2$ + 3P$_1$ + 3ADP $\dashrightarrow$ NAD + H$_2$O + 3ATP	oxidative phosphorylation

FIGURE 7-5

MODES OF ATP SYNTHESIS

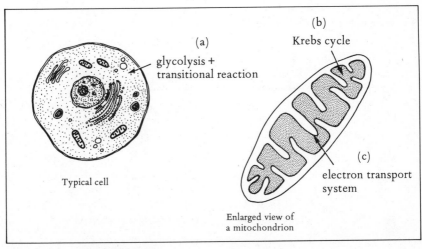

(a) glycolysis + transitional reaction

(b) Krebs cycle

(c) electron transport system

Typical cell

Enlarged view of a mitochondrion

FIGURE 7-6

CELLULAR LOCATIONS OF CARBOHYDRATE
METABOLISM

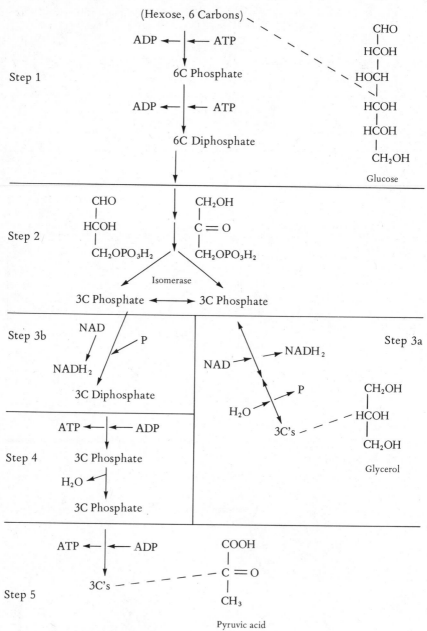

FIGURE 7-7

GLYCOLYSIS—"DISSOLUTION OF SWEETS"

known collectively as the *Krebs cycle.* Here the derivatives of glucose are further degraded to a molecule containing only one carbon atom, namely carbon dioxide. As with glycolysis very little ATP is generated directly by the Krebs cycle. During the Krebs cycle, however, certain energy-yielding oxidative reactions occur. It is these reactions that provide electrons for an oxidation-reduction system known as the *electron transport system.* The carriers for this system are located on microscopic projections on the inner mitochondrial membrane (Figure 7–6). It is here that the energy, which is made available as electrons travel from higher energy states to lower energy states, is stored by combining ADP with inorganic phosphate. With this overview in mind then, let's consider the various sequences in this carbohydrate refining process in more detail beginning with glycolysis.

GLYCOLYSIS Figure 7–7 presents a relatively simplified version of glycolysis, a series of reactions by which glucose, a six-carbon sugar (Hexose) is converted into energy and pyruvic acid and/or glycerol, both of which are three-carbon compounds. Pyruvic acid is an organic acid, while glycerol is an alcohol. The name glycolysis is derived from *glykus*—Greek for sweet, and *lysis*—Greek for dissolution or breaking down. Thus, glycolysis refers to the "dissolution of sweets." Glucose is a simple sugar, a hexose derived from the digestion of starch and plant juices. The process of converting glucose to pyruvic acid and/or glycerol begins at the cost of two ATP molecules, which are converted into ADP's. Thus a six-carbon diphosphate is formed during what we have called Step 1.

In Step 2, the six-carbon phosphate is split into two three-carbon phosphate compounds which differ slightly. However, there is an enzyme, triosephosphate isomerase, which can convert one of these three-carbon phosphate compounds into the other and vice versa. Recall that a three-carbon sugar is called a triose, and isomers are chemicals with a slightly different arrangement of the same atoms. The isomerase enzyme can change one form into the other. The structure of the two isomers in this case is shown in Figure 7–8.

In Step 3a, compound A is converted to glycerol and a molecule of NAD is reduced. Glycerol is an important subunit of fats and oils. Recall

$$
\begin{array}{ccc}
CH_2OH & & CHO \\
| & & \backslash \\
C = O & \text{and} & HCOH \\
| & & / \\
CH_2OPO_3H_2 & & CH_2OPO_3H_2 \\
\end{array}
$$

FIGURE 7–8

that NAD is a coenzyme which can be reduced by gaining hydrogens. These hydrogens can subsequently serve to reduce some other molecule(s).

In Step 3b, an additional phosphate is attached to isomer B forming a three-carbon diphosphate and a molecule of NAD is reduced. In Step 4 one of the phosphates is removed by attachment to an ADP, forming ATP by a substrate level reaction. In addition, the three-carbon phosphate molecule is oxidized. Subsequently in Step 5 the remaining phosphate is attached to ADP to form a second ATP and pyruvic acid.

When glucose is converted to two glycerol molecules, two ATPs are used initially and two $NADH_2$ are produced. Conversely, if glucose is converted to two pyruvic acid molecules, two ATPs are used, but four ATPs are produced as well as two $NADH_2$s. Thus the pathway to pyruvic acid is capable of yielding more energy directly in glycolysis, although the shorter path to glycerol is available if the cell needs that chemical to make lipids. Refer to Table 7–1.

TABLE 7–1
GLYCOLYSIS

Reactions	Net ATP's	$NADH_2$
Glucose ———— 2 Glycerols	−2	2
Glucose ———— 2 Pyruvic Acids	+ 2	2

ANAEROBIC REACTIONS The pyruvic acid and reduced NAD formed in glycolysis can undergo additional reactions in a variety of ways. Here we are concerned with *anaerobic* reactions, in actuality, *fermentation*. Pasteur stated, "La fermentation est la vie sans l'air"—Fermentation is life without air. More accurately anaerobiasis is life without air, and fermentation is the reduction of organic compounds under anaerobic conditions. Thus we are dealing with fermentation when we consider the use of reduced NAD to reduce pyruvic acid or a byproduct. In Figure 7–9 the central character is pyruvic acid.

The direct reduction of pyruvic acid by $NADH_2$ results in lactic acid, another three-carbon organic acid. This fermentation occurs for example in your muscles during exercise or work. When muscle cells consume oxygen at a rate faster than it can be supplied by the red blood cells an oxygen deficiency occurs. Instead of pyruvic acid and $NADH_2$ being used in aerobic systems, they combine producing lactic acid and fatigue. Thus under anaerobic conditions glycolysis still produces a net of two ATP, but the $2NADH_2$ produced during the glycolysis pathway are no longer available for future use. This fermentation also occurs in the souring of milk by bacteria to form yoghurt and the production of pickled cucumbers and sauerkraut. One bacterial culture that sours milk is called *Streptococcus lactis*.

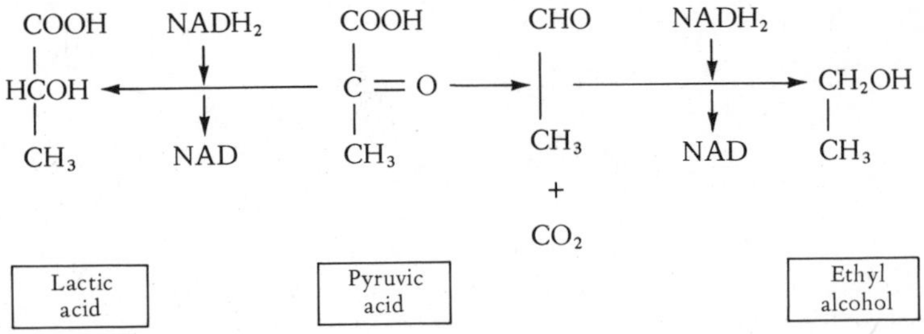

$$\underset{\text{Lactic acid}}{\boxed{\begin{array}{c} \text{COOH} \\ | \\ \text{HCOH} \\ | \\ \text{CH}_3 \end{array}}} \xleftarrow[\text{NAD}]{\text{NADH}_2} \underset{\text{Pyruvic acid}}{\boxed{\begin{array}{c} \text{COOH} \\ | \\ \text{C} = \text{O} \\ | \\ \text{CH}_3 \end{array}}} \longrightarrow \begin{array}{c} \text{CHO} \\ | \\ \text{CH}_3 \\ + \\ \text{CO}_2 \end{array} \xrightarrow[\text{NAD}]{\text{NADH}_2} \underset{\text{Ethyl alcohol}}{\boxed{\begin{array}{c} \text{CH}_2\text{OH} \\ | \\ \text{CH}_3 \end{array}}}$$

FIGURE 7–9

FERMENTATIONS INVOLVING PYRUVIC ACID

Streptococcus refers to the fact that the organism has a rounded shape (*coccus* = round) and occurs in chains (*strepto* = chain). *Lactis* refers to the production of lactic acid. One other bacterium involved in yoghurt production is called *Lactobacillus bulgaricus. Lactobacillus* refers to the fact that the organism is rod-shaped (*bacillus* = rod) and—*lacto*—makes lactic acid. The species name *bulgaricus* refers to the fact that the organism was originally found in a yoghurt from Bulgaria.

The ethyl alcohol fermentation is performed, usually, by yeast and, depending on the source of sugar and some other factors, results in beer, wine, whiskey, and so on.

TRANSITION REACTIONS The pyruvic acid formed in glycolysis can undergo reactions in addition to those described for anaerobic systems. The one of primary concern here, the transition reaction in the cytoplasm, is the means by which pyruvic acid is converted to an energy-rich two-carbon compound called *acetyl coA* or activated acetic acid. The acetyl coA is then available for a cyclical series of reactions, which yield considerable numbers of reduced coenzymes and a few ATPs by substrate phosphorylation. These reactions, which are found only in aerobic metabolism, are seen in Figure 7–10.

In transition, pyruvic acid (three carbons) is decarboxylated and NAD is reduced. In the process an energy rich sulfur bond is formed with an acetic acid (two carbons) molecule yielding the energy-rich acetyl coA (coenzyme A). The energy in this molecule is then available for the two-carbon acetyl coA and the four-carbon *oxaloacetic acid* to combine and form *citric acid,* a six-carbon compound.

KREB'S CITRIC ACID CYCLE The six-carbon citric acid then undergoes a series of molecular rearrangements which include *dehydrogenation* and *decarboxylation.* With the loss of a carbon as carbon dioxide (decarboxylation), ketoglutaric acid is the five-carbon compound produced. The

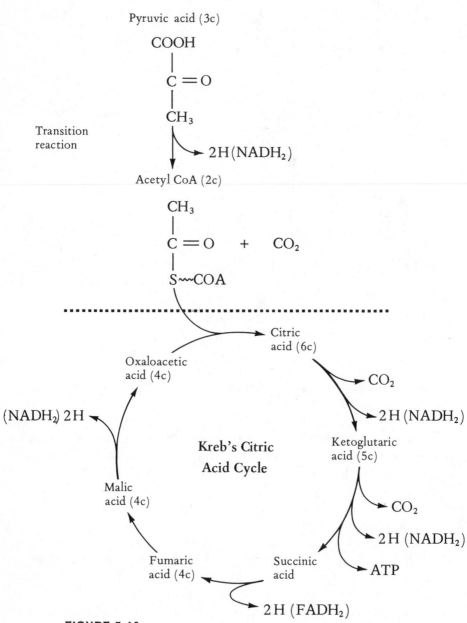

Pyruvic acid (3c)

Transition reaction

$$COOH$$
$$|$$
$$C = O$$
$$|$$
$$CH_3$$

2 H (NADH$_2$)

Acetyl CoA (2c)

$$CH_3$$
$$|$$
$$C = O \quad + \quad CO_2$$
$$|$$
$$S \sim COA$$

Citric acid (6c)

Oxaloacetic acid (4c)

CO_2

2 H (NADH$_2$)

(NADH$_2$) 2 H

Kreb's Citric Acid Cycle

Ketoglutaric acid (5c)

Malic acid (4c)

CO_2

2 H (NADH$_2$)

ATP

Fumaric acid (4c)

Succinic acid

2 H (FADH$_2$)

FIGURE 7–10
FROM GLYCOLYSIS THROUGH THE CITRUS ACID CYCLE

TABLE 7-2

TRANSITION REACTION AND KREBS
CITRIC ACID CYCLE—SUMMARY

Reactions	Net ATP's	$FADH_2$	$NADH_2$
Transition Reactions			
Pyruvic acid $\longrightarrow$ acetyl coA + CO_2	0	0	1
Krebs cycle			
Acetyl coA + Oxaloacetic acid $\longrightarrow$			
Oxaloacetic acid + 2 CO_2	1	1	3
Totals	1	1	4

lost hydrogens (dehydrogenation) are accepted by NAD and yield reduced NAD, $NADH_2$. Ketoglutaric acid is then subjected to a similar fate. It loses hydrogens to another molecule of NAD and a carbon as carbon dioxide. The resultant four-carbon compound is called *succinic acid*. In addition this reaction is also accompanied by a substrate phosphorylation producing a molecule of ATP. This is the only place where ATP is produced directly in the Krebs citric acid cycle. The four-carbon succinic acid now undergoes a dehydrogenation to produce the four-carbon *fumaric acid*. In this case the hydrogen acceptor is a different coenzyme, *FAD*. Next, fumaric acid is converted to the four-carbon *malic acid* by a molecular rearrangement. Finally malic acid is dehydrogenated, transferring hydrogens to a molecule of NAD and yielding the four-carbon oxaloacetic acid. With the formation of oxaloacetic acid, the Krebs citric acid cycle has completed one turn since the oxaoloacetic acid is once again available to combine with acetyl coA to form citric acid.

Every pyruvic acid in the transition reaction yielded one $NADH_2$ and the Krebs citric acid cycle yielded three $NADH_2$'s,.one $FADH_2$ and one ATP. These results are summarized in Table 7-2.

THE ELECTRON TRANSPORT SYSTEM Throughout glycolysis, the transition reactions and the Krebs Cycle, we have been removing pairs of hydrogen atoms from the intermediate molecules and combining them with other molecules such as NAD or FAD. Now let's consider how $NADH_2$ and $FADH_2$ are used to produce ATP energy in the *electron transport system*. First, what is the electron transport system, and how can it be applied to produce energy?

The electron transport system is a series of chemical intermediates located on the inner surface of the mitochondria. Each of these chemical intermediates is capable of accepting electrons and then passing these electrons to its neighbor. The chemical intermediates are arranged in descending order of total energy so that the electrons enter each successive chemical at a lower energy level releasing energy in the process. Because of the

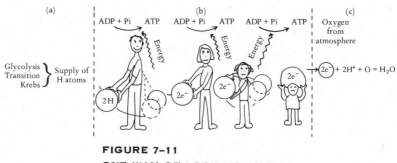

FIGURE 7–11

ONE WAY OF LOOKING AT THE ELECTRON TRANSPORT SYSTEM

decreasing energy progression, electrons will continuously move from one chemical in the series to another as long as two conditions are met:

1. There must be a source of electrons to begin the passing.
2. There must be an electron acceptor at the end of the chain to make room for the next electrons.

As Part a of Figure 7–11 shows, the first condition is met by the hydrogen atoms that are constantly being produced during glycolysis, the transition reaction, and the Krebs Citric Acid Cycle. Part way along the electron transport system the hydrogen atoms are stripped of their electrons and turned into hydrogen ions (Figure 7–11b). The electrons move along the chain and the ions move independently to the end of the chain where both meet the final electron acceptor, oxygen (Figure 7–11c). Thus, to meet the second condition, oxygen must constantly be supplied to the mitochondrion from the organism's environment for electron transport to proceed. Two hydrogens and their electrons combine with one atom of oxygen to form water. If this water is in excess of the cell's needs it will be eliminated by normal cell processes.

Now that we have introduced the electron transport system, we are prepared to analyze how this series of reactions is used to obtain energy. As the electrons join the first chemical in the series, they enter the compound at a relatively high energy level. The electrons then leave the first chemical and enter the second chemical at a lower energy level. As the electrons leave, the first chemical is transformed to its original state. The energy released in this reaction is used to combine ADP and phosphate to make ATP. A similar electron exchange and energy release occurs at each step in the electron transport system with the major differences being in the amount of energy released. At some stages energy is not released in a usable amount, resulting only in heat formation, while at other stages useful ATP is formed.

Let's consider the chemical reactions of the system in more detail (see Figure 7–12). Only the major electron acceptors are diagramed. The

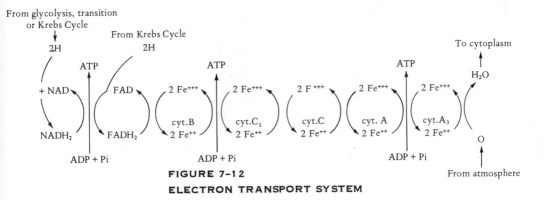

FIGURE 7-12

ELECTRON TRANSPORT SYSTEM

first electron acceptor in the series is NAD. As NAD is reduced by hydrogen, $NADH_2$ is formed. Almost instantaneously $NADH_2$ reacts with FAD, combining the FAD and hydrogen to form $FADH_2$. In the process NAD is regenerated, ready to accept the next pair of hydrogen atoms and the released energy is used to form ATP. $FADH_2$ then reacts with the first of a series of chemicals called *cytochromes* whose reactive portion in each case is an atom of iron (Fe) that is easily reduced then reoxidized. It is at this point that the hydrogen atoms are separated from their electrons. The electrons are passed from the iron of one cytochrome to the iron of the next cytochrome while the hydrogen ions follow separately. The electrons rejoin the ions and an atom of oxygen at the end of the chain to form water. This last reaction with oxygen is necessary in order to reconvert cytochrome oxidase to its usable oxidized form. As you can see in Figures 7–11 and 7–12, there are two more places in the electron transport sequence where the energy released is used to form ATP.

For the electron transport system to function, notice that only hydrogen and oxygen atoms need be supplied and only water needs to be removed. All other chemicals constantly present in the mitochondrion are not consumed, but rather, are constantly reconverted for use. The electron transport chemicals positioned in the membrane of the mitochondrion are rather like posts and barriers positioned in a pinball machine in order of decreasing total energy content (Figure 7–13). As the "ball" or electrons cross each scoring channel, one ATP is recorded. The barriers do not increase the score but are necessary to guide the ball down the energy gradient to the scoring channels.

The "posts" or chemicals are not altered in any permanent way and are equally ready to guide the ball and score more ATPs should more electrons from hydrogen become available to play with.

The electron transport system can be compared to a pinball game in yet another fashion. Some "balls" or electrons are propelled with more energy than others. We have just described those following the three ATP

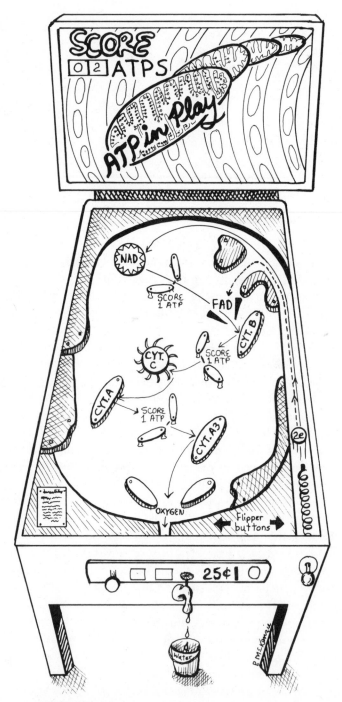

FIGURE 7-13

STILL ANOTHER WAY OF LOOKING AT THE
ELECTRON TRANSPORT SYSTEM

TABLE 7–3

SUMMARY OF ATP FORMATION FROM AEROBIC
CELLULAR METABOLISM IN AN EUCARYOTIC CELL

		Net ATPs
I. *Glycolysis*		
	2 ATP molecules utilized	
	4 ATP molecules produced by substrate phosphorytation	2
II. *Citric Acid Cycle*		
	2 ATP molecules produced by substrate phosphorytation	2

	ATP formed for each (2H)	Total ATP
III. *Oxidative Phosphorytation*		
A. Glycolysis		
2 –(2H) as NADH$_2$, however enter mitochondrion as FADH$_2$	2	4
B. Transitional Reaction		
2–(2H) as NADH$_2$	3	6
C. Citric Acid Cycle		
6–(2H) as NADH$_2$	3	18
2–(2H) as FADH$_2$	2	4
		32

Therefore:		
Net ATPs formed from one molecule of glucose in the presence of oxygen is		(36 ATP)

path. However, as we discussed earlier in the chapter, at one point in the Krebs Citric Acid Cycle electrons are released from a lower energy compound and first strike the FAD post following the two ATP path (dotted line, Figure 7–13). These last electrons can therefore, be used only to form two ATPs instead of the three ATPs formed by the higher energy electrons. This relationship can best be seen by comparing the positions of NADH$_2$ and FADH$_2$ in both Figures 7–12 and 7–13.

SUMMARY OF ATP PRODUCTION   We have now discussed all major sequences of reactions in carbohydrate (sugar) metabolism and are ready to briefly summarize the production of ATP from each sequence both during aerobic and anaerobic conditions. Results are summarized in Table 7–3. Of the three processes listed, only glycolysis may proceed anaerobically. Thus, anaerobically only a net of two ATP can be produced and those are from substrate level phosphorylations. Recall that the hydrogen atoms released during glycolysis are consumed during lactic acid or alcohol formation and are, therefore, unavailable to the electron transport system under anaerobic conditions. All remaining sequences of reactions listed only occur aerobically.

As the table demonstrates, aerobic metabolism produces far more ATP than anaerobic metabolism. Aerobically four ATP are produced by substrate level phosphorylations—two during glycolysis and two during the Krebs Cycle. In addition, *eucaryotic cells* produce thirty-two ATP by oxidative phosphorylation using the electron transport system. Thus, aerobically eucaryotic cells produce a net of thirty-six ATP compared with only a net of two ATP produced anaerobically. Obviously cells produce energy more efficiently in the presence of oxygen.

In the recent past all cells were thought to net thirty-eight ATP aerobically instead of thirty-six ATP. At present only *procaryotic cells* such as bacteria or blue green algae are still thought to produce a net of thirty-eight ATP. The discrepancy occurs in the ATPs produced from the hydrogens released during glycolysis. Glycolysis occurs free in the cytoplasm of cells while the hydrogens are used inside the mitochondria of eucaryotic cells. Energy is lost moving the hydrogens through the mitochondrial membranes and the hydrogens enter the transport system as $FADH_2$. Procaryotic cells, however, do not have mitochondria and this energy loss does not occur.

PROTEINS AND LIPIDS AS ENERGY SOURCES

So far, we have only been discussing the role of sugar in energy production. However, with diet crazes that include high protein–low carbohydrate diets, it is becoming increasingly obvious to the layperson that alternative energy sources of protein or fat may be utilized. How are these alternate chemicals metabolized to produce ATP?

Breakdown products of fats and proteins either form, or can be modified to form, intermediate chemicals in the carbohydrate utilization pathway. Several of these chemicals are shown in Figure 7–14.

Fats can be broken down into glycerol and fatty acids. Glycerol is a three-carbon compound that can readily enter the glycolytic pathway and can aerobically net seventeen ATP. Fatty acids are composed of long carbon chains that can be broken down two carbons at a time to form acetyl-coA. The two-carbon compound of the transitional reaction can be aerobically metabolised to produce twelve ATP. Since each molecule of fat can produce dozens of two-carbon compounds, it is no wonder that fats are known to contain vast stores of energy. In this respect they can be compared to using supreme gasoline in your race car instead of regular—you get more power per amount of fuel with fat than with carbohydrate.

If fat is supreme gasoline and carbohydrate regular, then proteins must be the least efficient unleaded variety of fuel. Proteins too can be modified to form intermediates of carbohydrate metabolism, sometimes, solely by removing the amine group. For example, the amino acid

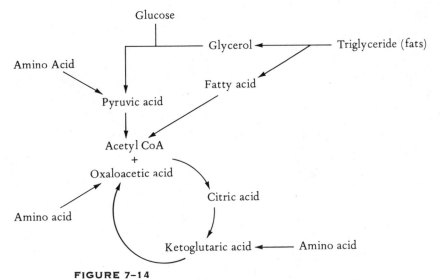

FIGURE 7-14

THE INTERRELATIONSHIP OF CARBOHYDRATES, FATS, AND PROTEINS IN ENERGY METABOLISM

$$H_2N - \underset{CH_3}{\overset{COOH}{\underset{|}{C}}} - H + H_2O + NAD \longrightarrow \underset{CH_3}{\overset{COOH}{\underset{|}{C}}} = O + NH_3 + NADH_2$$

L-alanine   Pyruvic acid

FIGURE 7-15

L-alanine (Figure 7–15) can be readily converted to pyruvic acid. Figure 7–14 indicates several other places where amino acids readily enter carbohydrate metabolic pathways to produce energy.

Note in each case that after deamination of the amino acid, the remaining chemical intermediate is not always capable of yielding as much ATP as a molecule of sugar or a molecule of pyruvic acid. Thus proteins have the lowest usable power yield of the three kinds of foodstuffs (refer to Figure 4–2).

SUMMARY In this chapter we have defined energy as the ability to do work and have identified ATP as the energy currency of all cells. We have identified carbohydrates as the main source of energy in cells but have shown how fat or protein may be used as an alternative. Energy production was shown to be far more efficient aerobically than anaerobically, with the greatest energy production coming from oxidative phosphorylation in the electron transport system. In the next chapter we will see some ways this energy is used to carry on life processes within the cells.

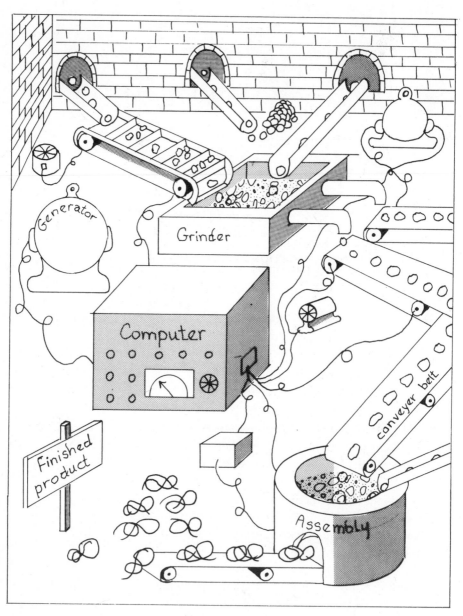

FIGURE 8–1
THE CELL AS A FACTORY.

Chapter 8
BUILD UP
Protein Synthesis and
Control of Enzyme Activity

In the last chapter you were lead through the series of "plays" by which the cell made available a usable supply of energy in the form of ATP. The mere production of energy, however, would be analogous to stalling a basketball game by merely dribbling and passing the basketball. Possession of the ball is a necessary requirement; but, unless the ball is shot at the basket no scoring can be done. So, too, in a cell, energy must be available, but it must also be utilized if the cell is to accomplish its goals.

WHY PROTEIN SYNTHESIS One way the cell uses or expends available energy is to anabolize, or synthesize, large molecules from smaller building blocks. In this, the final chapter, therefore, we have chosen to concentrate on how the cell manufactures and controls the production of one specific class of molecules, the proteins, which we see being assembled in our opening cartoon. Why proteins and not some other class of molecules? Earlier in the book we stressed the key roles played by proteins in various cell functions by labeling them as the top scorers of our molecular team of life. There is, however, a more basic, or fundamental, reason. The cell's overall "game plan" or blue print of activity is found in its genetic, or informational, material, which has been previously identified in Chapter 4 as DNA. But how is the plan of the game translated into the activity of the game, that is, how does the DNA actually direct the cell's activities? One way to approach this question is to consider some mistakes in the normal game plan known as genetic diseases. Several of these diseases along with their effects and causes are listed in Table 8–1.

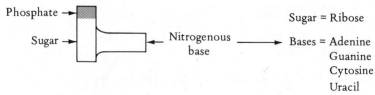

FIGURE 8-2

POSSIBLE COMPONENTS OF AN RNA NUCLEOTIDE

TABLE 8-1

SELECTED PROTEIN ABNORMALITIES

Disease	Effect	Cause
Sickle-cell Anemia	General Weakness	Abnormal Hemoglobin
Cretinism	Thyroid Malfunction	Absences of Enzyme deiodinase which normally catalyzes the removal of iodine from iodotyrosine
Galactosemia	Liver Enlargment; Galactose in blood	Absence of enzyme p-galtransferase which catalyzes transformation of galactose to glucose

Notice that in each case listed, the mistake has prevented a normal protein from being synthesized, and each malfunctioning protein is in turn responsible for the other effects noted. The message then is that each functional unit of DNA, called a gene, influences the play of the game by directly controlling the synthesis of a particular protein.

Our next question, therefore, is just how does the gene accomplish this synthesis of a specific protein? In our cartoon of the factory (Figure 8-1) the DNA is located in the computer that represents the cell's nucleus. Protein synthesis, however, occurs in assembly areas out in the cytoplasm called ribosomes. In a sense then, the DNA is like a coach on the sidelines who has to send information out to the field of play. The coach can send in a new player with directions for a play. But how does DNA get its information from the nucleus to the cytoplasm? This process, too, requires a messenger, and the messenger in this case is a second kind of nucleic acid known as ribonucleic acid, or more specifically as *messenger RNA* (m-RNA). Obviously the new player can verbally receive and transmit the coach's instructions for a play to the team on the field. But how is the m-RNA

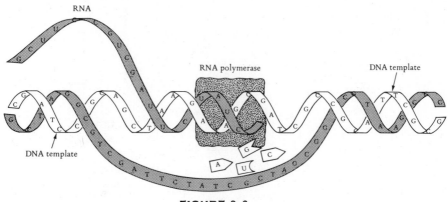

FIGURE 8–3
TRANSCRIPTION

molecule able to transmit directions from DNA to the protein assembly plants—the ribosomes? The answer lies in the manner in which this m-RNA is itself synthesized or made.

RNA SYNTHESIS—TRANSCRIPTION   As you may recall from Chapter 4, the basic building blocks of all nucleic acids are nucleotides. An individual nucleotide, as shown in Figure 8–2, has three components: a phosphate group, a sugar (which in RNA is ribose), and a nitrogenous base (which in RNA can be either adenine, guanine, cytosine or uracil).

The critical point, however, is the order in which these individual nucleotides are linked together to form a functional RNA molecule. This process is known as *transcription* and it can take place only in the presence of a DNA molecule. The DNA is not only a passive participant; rather, one of its two strands acts as a template or pattern for determining the sequence in which RNA nucleotides are linked together. Figure 8–3 shows the transcription process at work.

As you follow the two strands of DNA in from the far left, you can see that they uncoil, allowing the top strand to act as a template for RNA synthesis. In the center of the diagram a joining enzyme known as RNA polymerase is shown linking additional nucleotides to the growing chain of RNA. Notice, however, that the base sequence of the newly synthesized RNA is complimentary to the DNA strand being transcribed. For example, every place a guanine is present in the DNA strand, a cytosine is incorporated into the growing RNA chain. Likewise, an adenine is incorporated

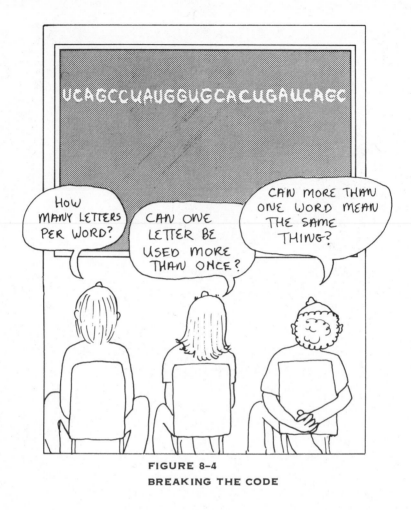

FIGURE 8-4
BREAKING THE CODE

into the RNA where thymine is present in the DNA, as is guanine for cytosine, and uracil for adenine. Synthesized in this way, therefore, the m-RNA molecule contains a base sequence, which intimately reflects the base sequence of a DNA molecule, or gene. Thus the information required for the synthesis of a new protein is passed from the DNA to the ribosome coded in the form of a linear sequence of bases in the m-RNA molecule.

THE GENETIC CODE What then is the language of the code? As our cartoon in Figure 8-4 indicates, the language contains only four letters in its entire alphabet, with each letter corresponding to one of the four different bases found in RNA. The first problem for the decoder, therefore, is to determine how many letters represent one code word. Recall that the purpose of the code is to specify the synthesis of a specific protein, and proteins are composed of linear chains of 22 different kinds of amino acids. The language must, therefore, have at least 22 code words.

Since there are only four letters in the language, a single letter code would allow for only four words. Likewise, code words containing two letters would allow for a total of only 16 different words—still not enough. If, however, each code word were to contain three letters, there is the possibility of 64 words—a more than ample number to code the 22 naturally occurring amino acids. Although words containing more than three letters could theoretically be possible, researchers have in fact demonstrated that each code word does contain three letters per word and is, therefore, *triplet* in nature. Moreover, as outlined in Table 8–2, they have been successful in determining the sequence of each code word.

Notice from the table that two code words, or *codons,* stand for the amino acid phenylalanine, namely UUU or UUC. Also the amino acid leucine is coded for by any one of six different codons: UUA, UUG, CUU, GUC, CUA, and CUG. Since more than one code word exists for many of the amino acids, the code is said to be *degenerate.* However, because no one codon can be used to code for more than one amino acid, the code is not considered to be *redundant.* The English language in contrast is redundant. One can, for example, *wind* a clock and also be blown by the *wind.* Or you can read that "the *lead* that led to the arrest of the suspect was the *lead* pipe found in the kitchen." The genetic code, however, does share another characteristic with the English language in that each letter in a sentence such as this one and each base in the genetic code is read only once: that is to say that the code is *nonoverlapping.*

TABLE 8–2

THE GENETIC CODE

1st base	Middle Base							3rd base
	U		C		A		G	
U	UUU UUC	Phenyl- alanine	UCU UCC	Serine	UAU UAC	Tyrosine	UGU UGC	Cysteine	U C
	UUA UUG	Leucine	UCA UCG		UAA Terminator UAG Terminator		UGA Terminator UGG Tryptophan		A G
C	CUU CUC CUA CUG	Leucine	CCU CCC CCA CCG	Proline	CAU CAC	Histidine	CGU CGC CGA CGG	Arginine	U C
					CAA CAG	Glutamine			A G
A	AUU AUC AUA	Isoleucine	ACU ACC ACA	Threonine	AAU AAC	Asparagine	AGU AGC	Serine	U C
	AUG	Methionine	ACG		AAA AAG	Lysine	AGA AGG	Arginine	A G
G	GUU GUC GUA GUG	Valine	GCU GCC GCA GCG	Alanine	GAU Aspartic GAC Acid		GGU GGC GGA GGG	Glycine	U C
					GAA Glutamic GAG Acid				A G

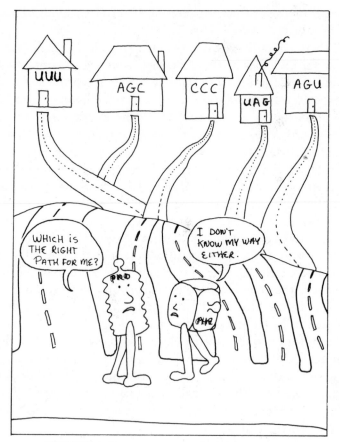

FIGURE 8–5A
HOW DO WE GET FROM HERE TO THERE?

Up to this point we have seen how the coach, DNA, is able to get a message out to the playing field by acting as a *template* for the production of m-RNA in the process known as transcription. Moreover, the message itself is locked into the triplet code expressed by the linear sequence of m-RNA bases. What remains now, therefore, is to see how this message is put into action on the playing field, that is, how the information contained in the m-RNA is translated into the production of a protein on the ribosomes—a process which is aptly referred to as *translation*.

PROTEIN SYNTHESIS—TRANSLATION The synthesis of a specific protein requires the joining together of specific amino acids in a certain special order, which, as we have seen, is dictated by the specific code sequence in the messenger RNA molecule. As our cartoon in Figure 8–5a indicates, however, the amino acids themselves are unable to interpret the

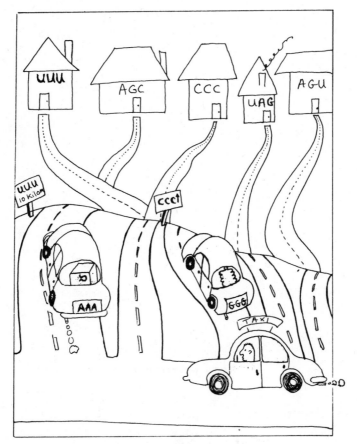

FIGURE 8–5B
CATCH A CAB

code, that is, they are unable to bond directly to their specific codons. As Part b of this figure shows, they must be carried to or matched-up with their respective code words by a class of "taxi" molecules known appropriately as *transfer RNAs* (t-RNA). This is possible because each kind of t-RNA has a three-base sequence, called an *anticodon,* which matches up with one particular triplet codon on the m-RNA (see the license plates of our t-RNA "taxis" in Figure 8–5b). The one critical factor that remains, however, is to insure that each amino acid gets into its appropriate taxi, that is, that an amino acid such as proline attaches to the t-RNA whose anticodon is complimentary to the m-RNA codon for proline. This is assured by the presence of specific taxi dispatchers who match up the appropriate amino acids with their particular t-RNAs. The dispatchers in the analogy are actually a group of enzymes with each enzyme having specific binding sites for a particular amino acid and its own special t-RNA.

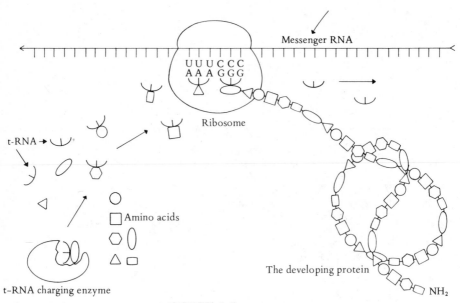

FIGURE 8–6
PROTEIN SYNTHESIS

At this point then we are prepared to review the execution of the play whereby a protein is synthesized. We will do this by referring to Figure 8–6. The code carrying m-RNA has left the nucleus and becomes attached to the ribosome. In the cytoplasm, specific amino acids have paired with their appropriate t-RNAs and are ready to be carried to the ribosome. Notice in the figure that the growing protein is attached to the t-RNA whose anticodon (GGG) is complimentary to the appropriate triplet on the m-RNA, namely CCC. Notice also that the next m-RNA codon UUU is being approached by the t-RNA bearing the complimentary anticodon AAA and that this t-RNA is carrying its specific amino acid, which is Phe (phenylalanine) in this case. Since no other t-RNAs will recognize this particular codon, Phe is the only amino acid that will line up on the ribosome at this particular position; hence the specificity. Moreover, once the amino acid is brought into place, it is positioned so that with the expenditure of some energy it can bond by a peptide bond to its adjacent amino acid, thus lengthening the growing protein molecule. In subsequent events the m-RNA moves along the ribosome thereby exposing the next specific codon, which will in turn be recognized by a specific t-RNA carrying its own specific amino acid. This process continues until the entire message has been read and all of the appropriate amino acids have been linked together by peptide bonds. The end product, therefore, is an intact protein

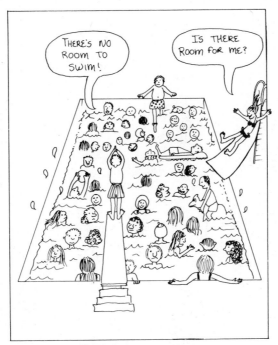

FIGURE 8-7
NO ROOM TO SWIM!

whose sequence of amino acids has ultimately been dictated by DNA through an m-RNA intermediary.

We have seen how one gene can code for one specific protein. In the human cell, however, there are well over a million individual genes. If each of these genes were to be transcribing all of the time, millions of different kinds of proteins would be coming off the assembly line continuously. As the cartoon of the crowded swimming pool (Figure 8-7) shows, it is unlikely that there would be room in the cell for all the possible proteins at one time.

LEVELS OF CONTROL   Since many of the proteins are enzymes that control the reactions of catabolism and anabolism, the cell must have mechanisms for regulating the production and/or activity of these enzymes. Basically these controls operate at one of two general levels. One level of control involves the transcription process of protein synthesis described earlier in this chapter. Remember, the information is transcribed into the messenger RNA for protein synthesis. At this level of control, the enzyme protein is either made or not made, depending upon whether the transcription process is allowed to occur.

The second general level of controlling enzymes occurs wherever the enzymes function. This may be in the cytoplasm, in membranes, or in the

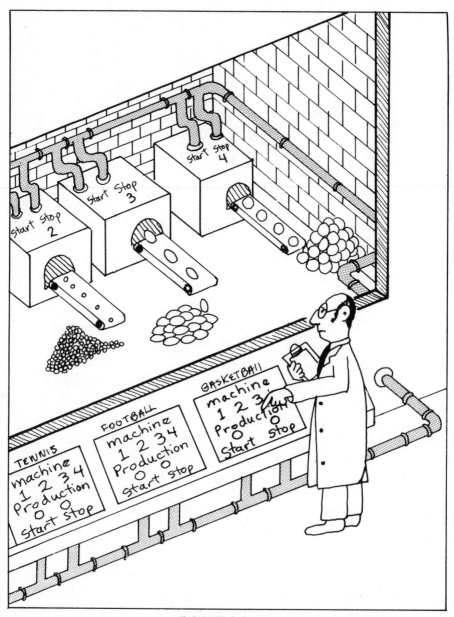

FIGURE 8-8
THE OPERATOR

nucleus. What is common to this level of control is that an enzyme is prevented from performing activity on a particular substrate. Thus we have chosen to call this the *substrate level* of enzyme control.

In the *transcription level* of control, regulation can occur in one of two ways, either *repression* or *induction.* Repression involves *stopping* the production of m-RNA for enzymes that are usually synthesized. Induction involves *beginning* the production of m-RNA for enzymes that are usually not synthesized. Inductible enzymes are needed only when a particular substrate is available. Both repression and induction are explained by what is called the *operon* model for control of transcription (see Figure 8–8).

Let's imagine someone, an operator, running a computer that produces instructions for each of several machines to make baseballs, footballs, basketballs, or tennis balls. This company has not had much marketing success for its tennis balls, but the other balls sell very well. Every time a machine is to make a particular batch of balls, instructions must come from the computer. Since baseballs, footballs, and basketballs sell so well, machines are fed these instructions automatically so that sometimes two machines can make one or another of these items. These items are subject to repression control. If baseballs began to accumulate in the warehouse, beyond anticipated needs, this would signal the operator to stop making instructions for baseballs and he would flip the appropriate switch. The tennis balls represent an inducible condition. The switch for these instructions is kept in the off position until a customer's order signals the operator to turn it on. Once the order is complete, the switch is flipped off.

In the case of repressible enzymes, the signal to stop transcription comes from the product of the enzyme activity. Let's suppose that the path in glucose catabolism from triose to pyruvic acid is under repression control. In this instance a build up of pyruvic acid would act as the signal to a gene called the operator. This operator gene would then cause transcription of the appropriate m-RNAs to cease. When the concentration of pyruvic acid decreased to some reasonable level, repression would be stopped by removal of the signal.

Probably the best known example of induction is the formation of the enzymes necessary to begin catabolism of lactose by *Escherichia coli,* a very common bacterium. When this organism is grown on media lacking lactose, it will not make any of the necessary enzymes. Now grow it on a medium with lactose, and that sugar signals the operator gene to turn on transcription of the appropriate m-RNAs. When the lactose has been metabolized, the switch is flipped off. Induction and repression are a way to allow a cell to function without the accumulation of excessive and unnecessary enzymes.

Repression serves as a rather coarse control of enzyme activity. A finer control is exhibited at the substrate level by a process called *feedback inhibition.* In this control mechanism enzyme synthesis is not affected,

(Part 1)

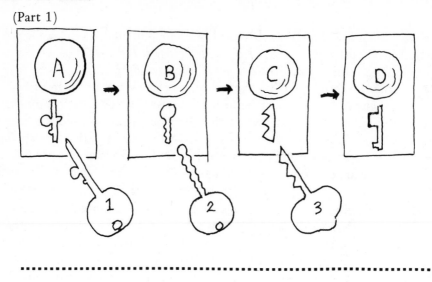

(Part 2)

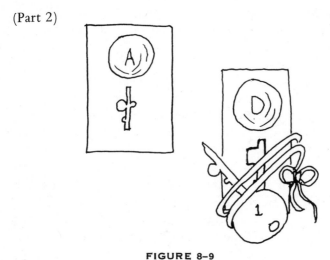

FIGURE 8–9
FEEDBACK INHIBITION

only the activity of a key enzyme in a particular pathway. In our hypo-
thetical metabolic pathway (Figure 8–9) compound A is changed to compound D. Using the lock and key analogy to demonstrate enzyme specificity (refer to Chapter 6 for review), you can see that the locks (substrates)
A, B, and C are slightly different, and so are the keys (enzymes) 1, 2, and
3 (Figure 8–9, Part 1). In this particular pathway, compound D would be
the end product of that series of reactions. In feedback inhibition, when
the end product accumulates above a certain concentration, that end product can attach to the first enzyme, key #1, and stop its activity (Figure
8–9, Part 2). The end product appears to change the shape of the enzyme,

and thus the substrate can no longer fit properly and gain access to the active site. We know that the synthesis of some amino acids is subject to feedback inhibition. Excess amino acid as end product stops the pathway until the amino acid may be used in protein synthesis, for example. Then when the concentration drops, inhibition is stopped and the pathway is back in business.

This, then, is the game cells play. We sincerely hope that our use of cartoons and analogies has helped you through some fairly complex material. We hope you have learned something about metabolism and maybe even enjoyed some of the process, for in the words of Sherlock Holmes, it is "Elementary" . . . to the study of physiology, pharmacology, microbiology, and many other -ologies.

Self-Test

1a. The ability to do work, that is, move a force through a distance is defined as:

   a. fuel
   b. catabolism
   c. energy
   d. catalysis
   e. none of the above

   b. Which of the following is a process that does not require energy?
   a. movement
   b. nerve impulse transmission
   c. synthesis
   d. diffusion
   e. secretion (export)

2. Which of the following *is not* a reason for the appropriateness of ATP as a cell's energy currency?
   a. It is present in large quantities in the food we consume.
   b. It can be readily made by cells from other foods that are eaten.
   c. It is readily available in all cells.
   d. When broken down it releases a large amount of energy.
   e. None of the above is a reason.

3. The mode of ATP synthesis during which an energy-rich food intermediate is further decomposed with the energy being utilized to bind a phosphate group to ADP is known as:
   a. substrate level phosphorylation
   b. oxidative phosphorylation

4. The following reaction sequences are involved in the production of ATP utilizing a carbohydrate source. For each of these reaction sequences, identify where in the cell each occurs:

   1. glycolysis
   2. transition relation
   3. Krebs cycle

   a. cell membrane
   b. cytoplasmic fluid
   c. mitochondrion
   d. nucleus
   e. lysosome

5a. Which of the following is not a reactant in glycolysis?
   a. glucose
   b. glucose phosphate
   c. 3 carbon phosphate
   d. ATP
   e. succinic acid

b. Triose phosphate isomerase controls the conversion of a six-carbon phosphate to a six-carbon diphosphate.
   a. true
   b. false

c. In the conversion of glucose to two molecules of pyruvic acid, two molecules of ATP are gained after subtracting two that are produced for the two that are consumed during glycolysis.
   a. true
   b. false

d. For each three-carbon phosphate that is converted to a three-carbon diphosphate, two molecules of reduced NAD are produced.
   a. true
   b. false

6. Which of the following is not produced when reduced NAD is reoxidized?
   a. ethyl alcohol
   b. pyruvic acid
   c. lactic acid

7a. Which of the following is not a major reactant in either the transition reaction or the Krebs cycle?
   a. acetyl coA
   b. lactic acid
   c. pyruvic acid
   d. citric acid
   e. oxaloacetic acid

b. For one transition reaction and one turn of the Krebs cycle, how many carbon atoms are lost in the form of CO_2?
   a. 1
   b. 2
   c. 3
   d. 4
   e. 5

   c. For one transition reaction and one turn of the Krebs cycle, how many reduced NADs and FADs are produced?

     a. 4 NAD, 1 FAD
     b. 3 NAD, 2 FAD
     c. 2 NAD, 3 FAD
     d. 1 NAD, 4 FAD
     e. None of the above combinations is correct.

   d. How many ATP are produced by the substrate level phosphorylation mode during one turn of the Krebs cycle?

     a. 1   b. 2   c. 3   d. 4   e. 5

8a. The proper sequence for the major acceptors in the electron transport system is:

     a. Cyt A, cyt A_3, cyt b, cyt c, FAD, NAD.
     b. NAD, FAD, cyt A, cyt A_3, cyt b, cyt c.
     c. NAD, FAD, cyt b, cyt c, cyt A, cyt A_3.
     d. FAD, NAD, cyt b, cyt c, cyt A, cyt A_3.
     e. None of the above is correct.

   b. Which of the following electron transfers are accompanied by ATP production (more than one choice is possible)?

     a. NAD–FAD
     b. FAD–NAD
     c. cyt b–cyt c
     d. cyt c–cyt b
     e. cyt a–cyt A_3

   c. When NADH is the initial electron donor, three ATP are produced; but, when $NADH_2$ is the initial donor of electrons only two ATP are produced in the electron transport system.

     a. true
     b. false

9. When the number of ATPs produced are considered, anaerobic respiration is unquestionably a much more efficient process than aerobic respiration.

     a. true
     b. false

10a. Amino acids (proteins) can be metabolized to produce energy by first being converted into all *but one* of the following substances. Which one is it?

     a. pyruvic acid   c. ketoglutaric acid
     b. oxaloacetic acid   d. glucose

b. Fats can be utilized to produce energy by being converted directly
into pyruvic acid.
   a. true
   b. false

CHAPTER 8: BUILD UP

1. A gene is that unit of genetic information which controls the production of which one of the following?
   a. nucleotide
   b. amino acid
   c. codon
   d. protein
   e. ribosome

2. Match the description in the left hand column with the appropriate
   term in the right hand column as it applies to the genetic code.

   ____1. more than one code word for one   a. redundant
          amino acid   b. nonoverlapping
   ____2. each code word composed of three   c. degenerate
          nucleotides   d. triplet
   ____3. one code word to specify more   e. foreign
          than one amino acid
   ____4. each letter in the code used in
          only one code word

3. In order to form RNA, the DNA nucleotides initially separate. They
   then exchange sugars, ribose for deoxyribose, and finally unite again
   as RNA.
   a. true
   b. false

4. Demonstrate your knowledge of the process of translation by answer-
   ing true or false to the following statements.
   1. Protein synthesis occurs in the nucleus.
   2. The m-RNA codons are recognized by the anticodon regions of
      t-RNAs.
   3. The individual amino acids are carried to the site of protein syn-
      thesis by enzymes.
   4. The newly formed protein consists of amino acids interspersed
      with t-RNAs.

5. When the activity of an existing enzyme is altered, this is considered to be control at the level of transcription.
   a. true
   b. false

6. In an inducible system the operator gene is sensitive to a signal that says to shut down the production of certain gene products.
   a. true
   b. false

7. In a system exhibiting feedback inhibition a certain end product inhibits the activity of an enzyme in the biochemical pathway.
   a. true
   b. false

ANSWERS TO SELF-TESTS
SECTION ONE
RULES OF THE GAME

CHAPTER 1: THE BASICS: Atoms and Molecules

1a. atom: Smallest unit of matter
 b. element: A kind of matter that is composed of like atoms
 c. molecule: Two or more atoms bonded together; most molecules are basic units of compounds
 d. compound: Matter formed by the combining of two or more elements

2. All atoms have a centrally located nucleus that contains protons and usually neutrons. The nucleus is orbited by electrons located in energy levels.

3. a. proton

4. b. neutrons

5. 1. b; 2. d; 3. e; 4. b; 5. a

6. reduction; oxidation

7. b. structural formula

8. a. catalysts

CHAPTER 2: MORE BASICS: Acids and Bases

1. a. Acids and bases are commonly produced by living systems.
   b. Acids and bases can potentially harm living systems.

2. Acids are substances that increase hydrogen ion concentration when placed in water.

3. Bases are substances that increase hydroxyl ion concentration when placed in water.

4. increases

5. 1. a; 2. a; 3. b; 4. b; 5. a

6. 1. c; 2. a; 3. b; 4. d

7. b. false

8. A buffer is a chemical or system of chemicals capable of combining with free hydrogen ion and free hydroxyl ion to minimize all pH changes.

9. bicarbonate (HCO_3^-); hydrogen ion (H^+) from carbonic acid (H_2CO_3)

10. Your text listed hemoglobin (Hb). Many other proteins make good buffers as do some of the materials associated with bones, and special buffer systems like the phosphate buffer system.

SECTION TWO
THE PLAYERS

CHAPTER 3: ELEMENTS OF LIFE: Carbon, Hydrogen, Oxygen, Nitrogen, plus Water

1. hydrogen (49%); carbon (25%)

2. b, c, d—Carbon tends to form four strong covalent bonds with a variety of different elements. Moreover, it can share more than one pair of electrons with a given atom by forming a double or triple bond, and it can bond to other carbons to form rings and a long chain.

3. b. false. On the contrary, oxygen is an avid electron seeker, tending to strongly attract electrons.

4a. d. As statement c indicates, the water molecule is assymetrical with the two hydrogens positioned on the same side of the oxygen (see Figure 3–6).
 b. false. Hydrogen bonds are intermolecular forces acting between different water molecules.

CHAPTER 4: MOLECULES OF LIFE: Protein. Carbohydrate, Lipid, and Nucleic Acids

1a. true. Recall the general formula for carbohydrates is $C_n(H_2O)_n$ where n stands for the number of carbon atoms in the molecule.
 b. d. Carbohydrates contain a store of energy that can be readily utilized by the cell.

2. triose—3; tetrose—4; pentose—5; hexose—6

3. a. true. Glucose and galactose both have the molecular fomula $C_6H_{12}O_6$.

4. c. Oligosaccharides contain a few (2-9) sugar units joined together.

5. b. false. Dehydration synthesis is the joining of two molecules together by means of *removing* the components of a water molecule.

6. polysaccharide; storage

7. b. Lipids are organic molecules, which as a class are insoluble in polar solvents such as water.

8. glycerol; fatty

9. b. false. Phospholipids are suited to be structural components of the cell membrane because they have both polar and nonpolar ends. The polar ends are attracted to water and the nonpolar ends to each other so that they line up side by side forming a boundary.

10a. b. Proteins
 b. c. The bearers of genetic information are the nucleic acid.

11. All amino acids have an amino (NH_2) group and an organic acid (COOH) group in common. Each of them however has an additional group (called an R group), which distinguishes one amino acid from another.

12. 1. d; 2. c; 3. a; 4. b

13. b.

14a. false. Each nucleotide does contain a phosphate group and an appropriate nitrogen base. But the sugar component in DNA is *deoxyribose* not ribose.
 b. adenine—thymine
 guanine—cytosine

15.

	Number of strands	Sugar	Bases present
DNA	2	deoxyribose	adenine thymine guanine cytosine
RNA	1	ribose	adenine uracil guanine cytosine

SECTION THREE
THE PLAYING FIELD

CHAPTER 5: LAY OF THE LAND: The Animal Cell
Answer Key to Factory Quiz
  a. brick wall and floor
  b. space in the room
  c. conveyor belts and chutes
  d. assembly machine
  e. grinder
  f. generator
  g. computer

1a. growth, increase in size of the individual.
  b. reproduction, increase in numbers of individuals.
  c. heredity, transmit characteristics to offspring.
  d. metabolism, all chemical activities necessary for life.
  e. organization, necessary groupings of parts.

2. lipid; protein; proteins

3. Diffusion brings molecules of food materials.

4. b. passive

5. energy.

6. a. true

7a. phagocytosis—process by which some animal cells capture organisms.
  b. pinocytosis—process by which animal cells take in fluids and small particles.
  c. moving molecules against the gradient; that is, chemicals go from low to high concentration

8. 1. d; 2. f; 3. a; 4. g; 5. b; 6. e; 7. c

CHAPTER 6: WARMING UP: Metabolism and Enzymes

1. *Catabolism* refers to chemical reactions dealing with the breakdown of complex organic materials and the production of energy. *Anabolism* refers to chemical reactions dealing with the build up or synthesis of organic materials and requires energy.

2. d.

3. The enzyme has a particular three dimensional shape, which corresponds to the shape of the substrate to be changed. Only a particular substrate and the corresponding enzyme can put together properly to allow a change to happen.

4. d.

5. a. split carbohydrates into simple sugar
   b. split proteins into amino acids
   c. split lipids (fats & acids) into component parts
   d. join subunits into large molecule like protein, nucleic acid or polysaccharide
   e. remove hydrogen from a molecule
   f. remove ammonia from a molecule
   g. remove carbon dioxide from a molecule

SECTION FOUR
THE GAME

CHAPTER 7: BREAKDOWN: Catabolism and Energy

1a. c. energy
  b. d. Diffusion is a passive process that naturally tends to occur without an input of energy.

2. a. See statement b.

3. a. substrate level phosphorylation. Oxidative phosphorylation is coupled to the passing of electrons along the electron transport system.

4. 1. b;   2. b;   3. c

5a. e. Succinic acid is a reactant in the Krebs cycle.
 b. b. false. Triose phosphate isomerase controls the interconversion of two three-carbon phosphates.
 c. a. true
 d. b. false. *One* molecule of reduced NAD is produced for each conversion.

6. b. Pyruvic acid is the substrate in the reaction during which lactic acid is produced.

7a. b. Lactic acid is an end product in anaerobic respiration.
 b. c.
 c. a. 4 NADH; 1 $FADH_2$
 d. a.

8a. c.
 b. a. NAD–FAD; c. cyt. B–cyt. C; e. cyt. A–cyt. A_3
 c. a. true. The first ATP coupling reaction is bypassed when FAD is the initial electron donor.

9. b. false. When a molecule of glucose is oxidized aerobically 36–38 ATP are produced, while only 2 are produced via anaerobic respiration. ation.

10a. d.
 b. b. false. The glycerol component of fats is initially converted into a three-carbon phosphate and the fatty acid components are degraded to Acetyl CoA.

CHAPTER 8: BUILD UP: Protein Synthesis and Control of Enzyme Activity

1. d.

2. 1. c;   2. d;   3. a. Recall, however, that the genetic code is *not* redundant, that is, no codon specifies more than one amino acid; 4. b. nonoverlapping

3. b. false. The DNA strands unwind but the individual nucleotides do not separate. Rather one DNA strand acts as a template for the lining up of specific RNA nucleotides, which are then joined together due to the activity of the enzyme RNA polymerase.

4. 1. false. Protein synthesis occurs on the ribosomes in the cytoplasm.
   2. true.
   3. false. The amino acids are carried to the ribosomes by their specific t-RNAs.
   4. false. The sole function of the t-RNAs is to carry amino acids to the ribosome and line them up according to the information contained in the m-RNA codons. A protein contains amino acids joined to one another.

5. b. false. Controlling the activity of an existing enzyme is said to be control at the level of substrate. Transcriptional control is extended at the level of the m-RNA produced to code for a particular enzyme.

6. b. false. In an inducible system the operator gene is sensitive to a signal that turns on certain genes, thereby producing the m-RNA, which codes for a particular protein.

7. a. true.

Glossary

ACID A substance that increases the hydrogen ion (H^+) concentration in water.

ACTIVE SITE That portion of an enzyme which is actively engaged in either bond making or breaking.

ACTIVE TRANSPORT The movement of a material against a concentration gradient, that is, from a lower to a higher concentration.

ADENOSINE TRIPHOSPHATE (ATP) The molecule that can be used by the cell directly as its energy currency.

AEROBIC Taking place in the presence of oxygen (air).

ALCOHOL An organic molecule that has a polar—OH group as its identifying characteristic.

ALKALI A substance that increases the hydroxyl ion (OH^-) concentration in water; a base.

ALKALINE A solution that has a higher concentration of hydroxyl ions than hydrogen ions; a solution that is basic.

ALPHA HELIX A spiral structure with a repeating pattern; it is a natural configuration in many biological molecules such as DNA and proteins.

AMINO ACID The building blocks of proteins. There are 20 commonly occurring amino acids.

AMINO GROUP The NH_2 group that is characteristic of all amino acids. This group can be removed from an amino acid by forming the base ammonia (NH_3).

ANABOLISM Those metabolic reactions that result in the build up, or synthesis, of larger molecules.

ANAEROBIC Taking place in the absence of oxygen (air).

ANTIBODY Certain protein molecules produced by the body in response to foreign substances called antigens, which they neutralize.

ANTICODON A sequence of three bases in a t-RNA molecule that are complimentary to a specific m-RNA codon.

APOENZYME The protein portion of an enzyme.

ATOM The basic unit of an element; it cannot be divided by ordinary chemical means.

ATOMIC NUMBER   The number of protons contained in an atom.

ATOMIC WEIGHT   A number approximately equal to the sum of all of the protons and neutrons in an atom.

ATP   Adenosine triphosphate; the molecule used as the cell's energy currency.

BASE   A substance that increases the hydroxyl ion (OH^-) concentration in water; an alkali.

BOND   An attractive force between atoms or ions.

BUFFER   A chemical or system of chemicals capable of combining with either free hydrogen ions or free hydroxyl ions so as to minimize all pH changes.

CARBOHYDRASE   An enzyme that catalyzes the breakdown of carbohydrates.

CARBOHYDRATE   A group of organic molecules including the sugars and polysaccharides that structurally are hydrates of carbon. The simplest have the general formula $C_n(H_2O)_n$ and are energy storing molecules.

CARBOXYL GROUP   The organic acid functional group, $-COOH$. A hydrogen ion dissociates from this group accounting for its acidic properties.

CATABOLISM   Those chemical reactions that result in the break-down of large molecules into smaller ones.

CATALYST   A substance that can increase the rate of a chemical reaction without itself being consumed during the reaction.

CELL   The basic unit of life; the smallest structure capable of exhibiting all the characteristics of life.

CHROMOSOME   A body found in the nucleus of a eucaryotic cell, which contains hereditary information in the form of DNA molecules supported by structural protein.

CODON   A sequence of three bases in an m-RNA molecule, which codes for the incorporation of a specific amino acid into a growing protein molecule.

COENZYME   A small organic molecule that combines with a protein to form an active enzyme.

COFACTOR   A small molecule usually inorganic, which must be bound to the protein portion of an enzyme in order for it to be active.

COMPOUND   Matter formed by the combining of two or more elements; a compound has properties that differ from those of the elements composing it. Example: water, H_2O.

CONCENTRATION   The amount of a substance per unit volume.

CONCENTRATION GRADIENT   The uneven distribution of a material in space, that is, large amounts of a substance in one area and lesser amounts of the same substance in an adjacent area.

CONSTITUTIVE   Refers to a class of enzymes that are synthesized in fixed amounts regardless of environmental conditions.

COVALENT   A type of bond in which electrons are shared between atoms.

CYTOPLASM   The area of the cell between the plasma membrane and the nucleus, literally cell matter.

DECARBOXYLASE An enzyme that removes a carboxyl group, which can then be eliminated as CO_2.

DEAMINASE An enzyme that removes an amino group ($-NH_2$) from an amino acid.

DEGENERATE CODONS Two or more codons that specify the same amino acid.

DEHYDRATION SYNTHESIS A chemical reaction during which small molecules are joined together by removing the components of water, H^+ and OH^-.

DEHYDROGENASE An enzyme that causes the removal of hydrogens from a molecule. These enzymes are responsible for many biological oxidations.

DEOXYRIBOSE The five-carbon sugar (pentose) that is a structural component of DNA nucleotides.

DNA Deoxyribonucleic acid; the genetic material.

DIFFUSION The passive movement of a material from a region of higher concentration to a region of lower concentration; diffusion does not require an expenditure of energy.

DIPEPTIDE Two amino acids joined together by a peptide bond.

DISSOCIATION The ionization of a substance when placed in water. For example, when dissolved in water, hydrogen chloride forms hydrogen (H^+) and chloride (Cl^-) ions.

DOUBLE BOND A covalent bond in which two pairs of electrons are shared between the same two atoms.

ELECTROLYTE A substance in solution that will conduct an electrical current due to movement of ions.

ELECTRON A negatively charged, relatively weightless particle found in an energy level of an atom.

ELECTRON ACCEPTOR A molecule that, because of its greater affinity for electrons, receives them from another molecule; an oxidizing agent.

ELECTRON TRANSPORT SYSTEM A series of molecules located on the inner surface of the mitochondrion that are capable of accepting electrons and then passing these electrons along to neighboring molecules.

ELEMENT A substance composed of only one kind of atom.

ENDOPLASMIC RETICULUM A network of membranous channels in the cytoplasm of a cell. These membranes are involved with the synthesis and transport of macromolecules.

ENERGY The ability to do work, that is, to move a force through a distance.

ENERGY LEVEL A region surrounding the nucleus of an atom in which electrons are found.

ENZYME A protein molecule that acts as a catalyst, that is, speeds up the rate of a chemical reaction.

EQUATION A symbolic representation of a chemical reaction by which the nature and amounts of reactants and products are identified.

EUCARYOTE A cell or organism composed of cells that have a true nucleus, that is, one in which the genetic materials are enclosed by a nuclear membrane.

EVAPORATE To convert to vapor (gas) usually by the application of heat.

FAT A type of lipid composed of the alcohol glycerol and a number of fatty acids.

FATTY ACID An organic acid containing a long chain of carbon atoms bonded to hydrogen atoms; a component of fats.

FEEDBACK The ability of an end product of a reaction sequence to influence an earlier reaction in that sequence.

FERMENTATION The reduction of organic compounds under anaerobic conditions.

GENE A functional unit of the genetic material DNA; a gene generally contains the code for the production of a protein.

GLYCEROL An alcohol containing three —OH groups; a component of many lipids such as fats.

GLYCOLYSIS A series of reactions by which glucose is converted into energy and pyruvic acid.

GROWTH The ability of living things to increase in size.

HEREDITY The ability of living things to give their offspring their own characteristics.

HEXOSE A monosaccharide containing six carbon atoms, for example, glucose and galactose.

HIGH ENERGY BOND A bond that when broken releases a large amount of energy.

HYDRATE A compound formed by the addition of water or both its components, H^+ and OH^-.

HYDROGEN BOND A weak bond formed between a hydrogen atom that is exhibiting an apparent positive charge, and another atom such as oxygen that exhibits an apparent negative charge.

HYDROGEN ION A hydrogen atom minus its electron; H^+.

HYDROLYSIS The breakdown of a molecule into smaller subunits by the addition of the elements of water; the opposite of dehydration synthesis.

HYDROXYL ION The OH^- ion formed by removing a proton (H^+) from water.

INDUCIBLE ENZYME An enzyme that is produced only when a certain substrate (inducer) is present.

INDUCTION A control at the level of transcription by which certain genes can be stimulated to produce their particular m-RNAs in the presence of an inducer.

INORGANIC All chemical substances that lack carbon as a central atom.

ION A charged atom having either an excess or deficiency of electrons.

IONIC BOND An attractive force formed between a positively charged ion and a negatively charged one.

ISOMER Molecules that have the same number and kinds of atoms, but with different spatial arrangements of these atoms.

ISOMERASE An enzyme that controls the conversion of one isomer into another.

KILOCALORIE A measure of heat energy equivalent to the amount of heat required to raise one kilogram of water $1°$ C.

KREB'S CITRIC ACID CYCLE   The series of biological oxidations that yield carbon dioxide and a large number of reduced coenzymes.

LIPASE   A lipid splitting enzyme.

LIPID   An organic molecule such as a fat or oil, which is insoluble in water and greasy to touch.

LYSOSOME   A membranous sac found in the cytoplasm of a cell, which contains enzymes that digest or break-down large molecules; literally a digesting body.

MESSENGER RNA (m-RNA)   The molecule transcribed from DNA, which carries the code for a particular protein from the nucleus to the ribosomes.

METABOLISM   The sum total of all of the chemical reactions that take place in a cell or organism.

MICROORGANISMS   Extremely small organisms usually visible only with the aid of a microscope, for example, bacteria and yeast.

MINERAL   An inorganic substance that is often required by an organism in small amounts.

MITOCHONDRION   Membrane bound cytoplasmic compartment that contains the enzymes required to convert selected chemicals into energy; power house of the cell.

MOLECULAR FORMULA   A combination of chemical symbols and numbers used to indicate the number and kinds of atoms present in a molecule.

MOLECULE   The smallest unit of a compound that still retains the properties of that compound; the chemical combination of more than one atom.

MONOSACCHARIDE   A simple sugar that cannot be broken down further by hydrolysis.

NAD   Nicotinamide adenine dinucleotide; a coenzyme involved in many biological oxidation-reduction reactions.

NEUTRAL   1. Electrical—having no net charge. This state is achieved when the number of protons present equals the number of electrons.
2. pH—when the hydrogen ion concentration is equal to the hydroxyl ion concentration; pH 7.

NITROGENOUS   Pertaining to any chemical containing nitrogen; nitrogen-containing bases are essential components of nucleic acids.

NONOVERLAPPING CODE   Term used to indicate that each nucleotide in the genetic code is read only once, that is, forms a part of only one code word.

NONPOLAR   Having an equal distribution of charge; opposite of polar.

NUCLEIC ACID   Molecule composed of phosphate groups, sugars, and nitrogenous bases; the class of molecules that contains and transfers genetic information.

NUCLEOTIDE   The building block of a nucleic acid composed of a phosphate group, a five-carbon sugar, and a nitrogenous base.

NUCLEUS   The center or core of anything. 1. The cell structure that contains the genetic information. 2. The portion of an atom containing the protons and neutrons.

OLIGOSACCHARIDE   A carbohydrate that contains from two to nine simple sugar units, for example, the disaccharide maltose.

OPERON   A group of adjacent genes that operate in a coordinated fashion under the influence of a common operator gene.

ORGANIC   Historically, a substance produced by a living organism; a substance that contains carbon as a central atom. CO_2 is a rare exception.

OXIDATION   A chemical reaction that is accompanied by the loss of electrons.

OXIDATIVE PHOSPHORYLATION   The production of ATP by utilizing the energy made available by the oxidation of a coenzyme such as NADH.

OXIDIZING AGENT   A substance that accepts electrons from another substance.

PASSIVE TRANSPORT   The movement of a substance along a concentration gradient from high to low without the expenditure of energy.

PEPTIDE BOND   The bond  that links together two amino acids by joining the carboxyl carbon of one to the amino nitrogen of the other.

pH   A scale running from 0 to 14, which gives a measure of the hydrogen ion concentration; the higher the hydrogen ion concentration, the lower the value on the scale.

PHAGOCYTOSIS   Literally, cell eating; a means whereby cells can ingest large particles with the expenditure of energy.

PHOSPHOLIPID   A class of lipids that contains a phosphate derivative in place of a fatty acid, making them polar.

PINOCYTOSIS   The movement of fluid from outside of the cell to the inside by trapping it in small sacs of the lipid membrane.

PLASMA MEMBRANE   The boundary between the cell and its environment; a lipid bilayer with various proteins on and within the lipid layers.

POLARITY   Characterized by an uneven distribution of charges.

POLYMER   A large molecule formed by the joining together of many subunits; for example, a protein is a polymer composed of many amino acids.

POLYMERASE   An enzyme that joins subunits together to form a polymer.

POLYPEPTIDE   A compound formed by the joining together of two or more amino acids.

POLYSACCHARIDE   A compound formed by the joining of many simple sugar units together.

PROCARYOTE   A cell or organism that lacks a true nucleus, that is, one in which no nuclear membrane surrounds the genetic material.

PRODUCT   A substance that results from a chemical change.

PROTEASE   An enzyme that digests or breaks down protein.

PROTEIN   An organic molecule composed of many amino acids joined together.

PROTON   A positively charged particle located in the nucleus of an atom.

REACTANT   A starting material in a chemical reaction.

REDUCING AGENT   A substance that loses electrons to another substance thereby causing the second substance to be reduced, that is, to gain electrons.

REDUCTION   A chemical reaction in which electrons are gained.

REDUNDANT CODE   A code in which one code word has more than one meaning; the genetic code is not redundant, that is, each codon specifies only one amino acid.

REPRESSION   The ability of an end product to shut down the genes responsible for the enzymes that control the production of that particular end product.

REPRODUCTION   The ability of living things to increase their numbers.

RESPIRATION   The oxidation of fuel molecules such as sugars to yield useable energy in the form of ATP.

RIBOSE   The five-carbon sugar that is an essential component of ribonucleic acid.

RIBONUCLEIC ACID (RNA)   The class of nucleic acids that has ribose as its sugar component and uracil as one of its nitrogenous bases.

RIBOSOMES   Cytoplasmic granules, often associated with the endoplasmic reticulum, which serve as the site of protein synthesis.

RNA   See Ribonucleic Acid

SALT   A product of the reaction between an acid and a base.

SOLUBLE   Capable of being uniformly dissolved in a liquid.

SOLUTION   A uniform mixture in which a solute such as sugar is evenly dispersed in a solvent such as water.

SOLVENT   A substance, usually a liquid, that is capable of dissolving another substance.

SPECIFICITY   The ability to perform one particular reaction or type of reaction.

STABLE   Not easily decomposed; showing a decreased tendency to react.

STRUCTURAL FORMULA   A means of representing a molecule that shows the spatial arrangement of its component atoms.

SUBSTRATE   The substance acted upon by an enzyme.

SUBSTRATE LEVEL PHOSPHORYLATION   The decomposition of an energy rich food intermediate with the energy release used to drive the synthesis of ATP.

TEMPLATE   A pattern or guide used to shape or construct something; DNA is the template used to synthesize RNA.

TERMINATOR   A codon that signifies the end of a protein message.

TRANSCRIPTION   The synthesis of RNA using the base sequence in DNA as a template.

TRANSFER RNA   The class of RNA molecules that attaches to specific amino acids and carries them to the ribosomes as determined by the m-RNA codons.

TRANSITION REACTION   A reaction, occurring in the cytoplasm, by which pyruvic acid is converted to an energy rich two-carbon compound called acetyl CoA.

TRANSLATION   The synthesis of a protein on the ribosome. The particular amino acid sequence of the protein is determined by the code words present in m-RNA.

TRIOSE   A simple sugar containing three carbon atoms.

VITAMIN   Small organic molecules that function as cofactors necessary for the activity of many enzymes. As the name indicates vitamins are vital for life and must be included in one's diet.

Index